Simone Cave is the author of five international bestsellers on parenting and childcare. She was the health editor at the *Daily Mirror* for eight years and is now a freelance journalist covering nutrition, health, medical and parenting issues for national newspapers and magazines. Simone lives with her husband and three young children in London. www.yourbabyandchild.com

Dr Caroline Fertleman is consultant paediatrician at the Whittington Hospital, London. She also works at the Institute of Child Heath at University College London and has an honorary contract at Great Ormond Street Hospital for Children. Caroline has written several books on babies, toddlers and potty training. She lives in London with her husband and three children.

YOUR BABY
Week by Week

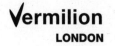

Simone Cave and
Dr Caroline Fertleman

Vermilion
LONDON

20 19 18 17 16 15 14 13

Published in 2007 by Vermilion, an imprint of Ebury Publishing

Ebury Publishing is a Random House Group company

Copyright © Simone Cave and Caroline Fertleman 2007

The Random House Group Limited Reg. No. 954009

Addresses for companies within the Random House Group can be found at www.randomhouse.co.uk

A CIP catalogue record for this book is available from the British Library

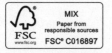

The Random House Group Limited supports the Forest Stewardship Council® (FSC®), the leading international forest-certification organisation. Our books carrying the FSC label are printed on FSC®-certified paper. FSC is the only forest-certification scheme supported by the leading environmental organisations, including Greenpeace. Our paper procurement policy can be found at www.randomhouse.co.uk/environment

Printed in the UK by CPI Group (UK) Ltd, Croydon, CR0 4YY

ISBN 9780091910556

Copies are available at special rates for bulk orders. Contact the sales development team on 020 7840 8487 for more information.

To buy books by your favourite authors and register for offers, visit www.randomhouse.co.uk

Please note that conversions to imperial weights and measures are suitable equivalents and not exact.

The information given in this book should not be treated as a substitute for qualified medical advice; always consult a medical practitioner. Neither the author nor the publisher can be held responsible for any loss or claim arising out of the use, or misuse, of the suggestions made or the failure to take medical advice.

To Lewis, Douglas, Harry, Tobias and Betsy

acknowledgements

We would like to thank Paul Johnson, Judy Cave, Alex Cave, Barbara Levy, Jo Carroll, Yiannis Ioannou, Debbie Cowen and Adrian Cohen, as well as health care professionals both at the Whittington Hospital and elsewhere.

contents

introduction

Everyone tells you that babies don't come with a manual. Well, maybe they're wrong because here it is. We've written *Your Baby Week by Week* to gently guide you through the incredible first six months of your baby's life. We aim to hold your hand during those stressful times when every cry will set your heart racing, and every snuffle send you running to the doctor.

Of course, we understand that parents are hungry for facts about their newborns – why are they awake most of the night, is their poo normal, and are they feeding properly? And yet we also realise how exhausted you'll be feeling. Even finding time to eat breakfast can be a struggle, so doing in-depth research on jaundice is the last thing you'll feel like. This is why we've given you all the facts you'll need for each week in the first six months of your baby's life and presented them in a simple, easy-to-follow format. Each chapter is broken into clear sections covering a full range of practical issues, from sleeping and crying, to nappies and when to call a doctor.

Beginning with week 0 when your baby is first born, we explain everything from how many wet nappies you can expect over 24 hours to how long your baby might sleep and cry for. We've tried to describe every possible event that can occur in that first week so have included detailed information about your midwife's visits, how to spot if your baby is dehydrated, and whether he is feeding properly. We've even put in a 'What's happening to mum' section which tells you, among other things, which day the baby blues are likely to kick in. This comprehensive detail continues throughout the book and each chapter tells you what you need to know for a particular week.

You'll notice that we always refer to the baby in the book as 'he'. This is simply because we, the authors, have five children between us, four of which are boys. We could just as easily have said 'she' and probably would have done if we'd had more daughters.

We know that small groups of mums with babies the same age gather up and down the country earnestly comparing notes about their tots. So we've given this book the reassuring voice of a good friend who is also an experienced mother, a consultant paediatrician, and just happens to have a baby who was born in the same week as yours.

THE PHILOSOPHY

While researching this book we noticed that baby experts fall into two main groups. There are those who recommend a strict routine with regular feeding and sleeping times, and those who emphasise the importance of following your baby's demands by ignoring the clock and letting your baby do what he wants to. Both of these approaches have a lot of advantages – and disadvantages – which is why we've taken a middle-of-the-road, best of both worlds approach. But it's important to point out that babies change so rapidly during the early months that guidance needs to adapt quickly too. Advice that is relevant for a two-week-old isn't necessarily suitable for a baby who is six weeks old. And this is where giving week-by-week advice comes into its own.

For example, during the first few weeks you definitely need to take more of an 'earth mother' approach, cuddling and feeding your baby around the clock. This is crucial to his development and it can actually be dangerous to only feed your baby at regular intervals at this stage because he could well end up dehydrated. Caring for your baby in this way allows you to be disorganised and chaotic in the early weeks, which will reduce your stress considerably. But if you continue this very relaxed, unstructured approach, you may find yourself exhausted if, at six weeks, your baby is still demanding to be fed every hour and refuses to sleep unless he is in your arms. That's why we've included a step-by-step sleep programme, giving tips relevant to a particular week, to help you eventually to get your baby sleeping through the night by six months.

We've also explained how to get your baby into a routine, but our approach is both gentle and realistic – we've made plenty of allowances for problems such as colic and unusually difficult babies. And throughout the book we've offered trouble-shooting advice to help you identify the exact reason why your baby may not be feeding or sleeping as expected.

We have strived against telling you what to do or giving hard and fast instructions and instead have adopted a gentler, advisory approach – after all he's your baby. A mother's instinct is extremely strong, and our intention is not to counter this but to reinforce it with the appropriate facts and information to give you the confidence to do what you know to be best for your baby.

HOW TO GET THE MOST OUT OF *YOUR BABY WEEK BY WEEK*

We know that you're busy and tired, so we've made it easy for you to find the information you need. Obviously you read the week appropriate to your baby's age, beginning with week 0 when he is born, week 1 when he is a week old, and so on. And you'll probably find yourself flicking through to future weeks to discover what lies ahead. Once your baby is born you probably won't be able to study this book from cover to cover – though of course if you're reading it while pregnant there's no reason why you can't use it to prepare yourself for motherhood.

There's no need to read every section in a chapter – just pick out the ones that seem relevant. So if you're worried about your baby's feeding then you'll turn straight to the feeding section and perhaps return another time to the sections on subjects such as washing or development.

Don't worry if your baby's progress doesn't seem to tally with the manual. Babies are far from an exact science; they are all vastly different so of course there will be variations between your baby and what we describe. This point is particularly applicable to the 'Development and playing' section, which covers physical and mental milestones your baby may have reached. The aim of this section is to be fun and to help you observe the tiny changes your baby will go through, such as when he stops keeping his hands in permanent fists. There's a small chance that this section may help to pick up problems, with your baby's hearing for example, but this isn't the main purpose. And we certainly don't want it to make you feel competitive or anxious in any way.

We've been careful to explain whenever there could be a problem if your baby doesn't reach a particular milestone, otherwise you must assume that your baby is perfectly normal but is just developing at his own speed.

If the topic or information you're looking for isn't covered in the particular week you're reading, you could always flick back or forward a chapter or two to see if you get a more detailed picture – also use the index at the back.

WEANING

You'll find that you get the most from *Your Baby Week by Week* by reading the week that is relevant to your baby's age. There's one possible exception and that is our step-by-step weaning programme, which we introduce at 17 weeks. A lot of mums won't want to start their babies on solids until they are older, and may well want to wait until six months before weaning. We've outlined the pros and cons in the book to help you decide when to start weaning your baby. Once you've made up your mind about at which age you're going to start, you simply begin at week 17, however old your baby actually is, then follow the advice through the subsequent weeks.

HEALTH AND SAFETY

When it comes to your baby's health, we've included the most common ailments in the 'When to call a doctor' section. Although do be aware that these illnesses may well occur in different weeks. We've put them in when we think they are most likely to occur. But as we've stressed throughout the book, you should always seek medical advice if you are concerned about your baby. The safety tips will also be relevant in various different weeks, but again we've put them in when we think they are most likely to be an issue.

WHO IS THE BOOK FOR?

As well as being essential reading for first-time parents – including dads – we also highly recommend this book for parents having their second, third or even fourth babies. Although you've done it all before and can change a nappy with lightning efficiency, looking after a new baby is a tremendous challenge however many children you've already got. And don't forget that with other children to look after you'll have even less energy than previously. So you'll find it useful to have the manual to hand to jog your memory about things like when your baby is supposed to start having three naps a day, for example, and how often you're supposed to be feeding him.

We sincerely hope that having *Your Baby Week by Week* to hand during those early months will prove invaluable and take a little of the angst out of looking after your new baby. As mothers ourselves, we certainly wish we'd had such a book when we first entered parenthood. It's only when you dare to stop worrying that you'll be able to relax and enjoy your baby to the full extent, in the knowledge that he's healthy and that you are doing the right thing as a parent. We believe that if you are armed with the relevant facts you will be vastly more confident as a parent and be able to tune in to your own instincts and your baby far more effectively.

week 0

Arriving home from hospital with your brand new baby is when reality kicks in for most new parents. For the past few days you've been cocooned by a safety net of medical staff, and now you're on your own it will probably dawn on you just how little you know about looking after a newborn baby.

But you're not quite on your own yet because the day after you leave hospital you'll get a visit from a community midwife. She will probably turn up unannounced, but don't worry about tidying the house or even getting dressed – she's there to help and won't judge you. The midwife will feel your tummy to check that your womb is contracting, and then take your pulse, blood pressure and temperature to rule out infection and problems resulting from the birth. She will ask how you are feeling both physically and emotionally, and make sure there are no problems with your breasts, whether or not you are breastfeeding. The midwife will also check your sanitary pad to make sure that any blood loss is normal and look at your legs to rule out blood clots, and finally she will check your stitches if you had them. She'll also answer all your questions and give any baby care help that she can – for example with breastfeeding.

As well as making sure that you are okay, your midwife will examine your baby. She'll weigh him, look at his cord stump, check the colour of his skin to rule out jaundice, and take his temperature. Your midwife will also give your baby a heel prick test on his seventh day. This involves taking a blood sample from his heel which may make him cry briefly. The blood is tested for phenylketonuria (PKU – a treatable metabolic disorder), hypothyroidism (a treatable thyroid disorder), sickle cell disease (a treatable blood disorder), MCADD (a treatable digestive disorder) and cystic fibrosis (a manageable lung and digestive disorder). Most of these conditions are rare but straightforward to treat if picked up early. You'll hear results within six weeks.

If you had a home birth, your midwife will leave a few hours after the birth, but return later that day or the next when you'll also get a visit from your GP to check your baby over.

Whether you had a home or hospital birth, your midwife will continue to visit for the next 10 days, probably every other day. She'll leave you a 24-hour telephone number so that you never feel completely on your own. It's natural to have dozens of worries this week, so don't hold back in speaking to your midwife however petty you think your concern may sound.

SLEEP

Total sleep required: *16–20 hours a day*
Pattern: *irregular*

Your baby will be exhausted from the birth, so on the first night you may well get a good sleep and a chance to recover from the birth. He is likely to sleep for up to 10 hours without wanting milk or needing his nappy changed. If you're in hospital, put some ear plugs in and make the most of it as this will be the last unbroken night's sleep for months.

Your second night with your new baby will probably be a very different story as his appetite kicks in, making him wake every hour or two for a feed. Newborns have no circadian rhythms – which regulate the body clock – so they don't get any sleepier at night.

Instead they will constantly nap and feed around the clock, oblivious to whether it is night or day.

Console yourself with the fact that newborns can't stay awake longer than about 90 minutes at a time, which means that if, say, you're finding it impossible to settle your baby at 4am, he'll drop off after an hour and a half at the most. It's normal for babies to sleep very erratically this week, so don't even think about sleeping patterns; the most he will sleep for is three hours at a time. Try to go with it, and don't get anxious about your own sleep deprivation – you'll almost certainly see a small improvement by the end of the week as your baby occasionally goes for longer between feeds. Feeling exhausted and fluffy-headed this week is normal and means that you are responding to your baby's needs. There are no quick fixes at the moment to get your baby to sleep for longer.

CRYING

Number of hours your baby may cry in a day: 1–3 is usual, but some babies can cry for up to 12 hours

You may be lulled into a false sense of security at the beginning of the week if your baby hardly cries and sleeps most of the time. This is nature's way of giving you and your baby a chance to recover from the birth. After a few days your baby will cry more and you'll probably have no idea why. You won't yet know him well enough to distinguish his different cries but there's a good chance he's crying because he's hungry. He's too young to cry from being overtired or because he's got a wet nappy. So whether you are breast- or bottle-feeding, offering him milk whenever he cries is your best chance of soothing him.

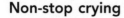

Non-stop crying

Some breastfed babies scream continually for hours on end any time from day two to day five because they can't get enough milk. Breastfeeding mothers produce colostrum for the first couple of days, a thick milk rich in antibodies and nutrients. The purpose of colostrum is to help protect your baby against infection. You only produce tiny amounts but this corresponds to your baby's appetite as he won't be especially hungry initially.

By about day three, colostrum is replaced by 'real' milk – which isn't as thick, but there is far more of it so your baby feels full and satisfied after a feed. But nature frequently gets the timing wrong and your baby may be ready for the 'real' milk before your body has started producing it. The result is that you have a very placid baby while you are in hospital, but almost as soon as you get home he starts screaming non-stop. This will go on until your milk starts flowing freely, which can take up to day five.

Naturally, it's distressing not being able to satisfy a hungry baby but do let him suckle often as this speeds up your milk reflex; sucking makes prolactin, a hormone that triggers your milk supply and also calms babies, so will hopefully give you a little peace.

While you are waiting for your milk to come through, you may be tempted to give your baby some formula milk. The main advantage is that this will stop him crying from hunger. The big disadvantage is that if you don't put your baby to your breast often enough, it could interfere with your milk production and delay your milk even more. But your baby won't starve – your midwife can give reassurance when she weighs him.

One compromise is to offer your baby a couple of ounces of formula when he seems especially distressed, then when he is calmer let him suck from the breast. Although some midwives would disagree with giving formula milk this early if you are trying to breastfeed, the odd emergency bottle is better than ending up back in hospital because your milk hasn't come through and your baby is desperately hungry and becoming dehydrated.

FEEDING

Total milk required: about 450–600 ml/15–20 oz a day
(30–90 ml/1–3 oz per feed)
Pattern: irregular, up to 12 feeds a day

During week one, your main goal should be to get feeding established. This can be challenging because new babies need to learn what to do and will seem a bit confused and clumsy whenever they are offered a breast or a bottle.

Do feed on demand, whether breast- or bottle-feeding. This is important because a newborn's stomach is very small, so he needs lots of little feeds. And current thinking is not to push a newborn into a four-hour feeding pattern because he will feel hungry on this regime.

Offer your baby milk every time he cries and forget about a regular feeding pattern for the moment. If you follow your baby's demands, feeding will be erratic. Sometimes he'll want to feed every hour, and then you might find that occasionally he'll go for four hours without food – don't let him go longer than this as his blood sugar will drop and he'll feel too sleepy to wake up and demand food.

You'll also find that your baby will want different amounts of milk at each feed, sometimes just 30 ml/1 oz, other times he may manage 90 ml/3 oz. If you're breastfeeding, you won't have any idea how much your baby is taking, but you will notice that feeds can vary in length from about five minutes to an hour.

Breastfeeding

The list of advantages of breastfeeding is endless and new reasons to breastfeed are being discovered all the time. Breastfed babies are less likely to suffer from respiratory infections, stomach bugs, allergies and diabetes than bottle-fed babies. They are also likely to have higher IQs and be less likely to get heart disease in later life. Other advantages of breastfeeding are that you will burn an extra 200 calories a day, which helps shed your pregnancy weight, you'll reduce your risk of breast cancer, and your baby's nappies won't be as smelly as a formula-fed baby.

But there is a real knack to breastfeeding and many women struggle. So although around 70 per cent of mums try to breastfeed their newborn in the first week, this plummets to 50 per cent in the second week. And just one in five babies are breastfed by the time they are six months old. We shall be looking at the reasons mums give up breastfeeding this week and next, and explaining how to solve these problems.

Why you may want to give up breastfeeding this week

You can't get started

If your baby seems to have 'lost' your nipple, tickle his upper cheek to coordinate his rooting reflex – new babies often root for the nipple in the wrong direction. You can also squeeze out a little milk by hand for him to smell.

You may also find that his arms are flailing, in which case tuck his lower arm (the one nearest to you) behind your back. You could also try swaddling him using a muslin cloth folded into a triangle. Wrap each corner over his arm and behind his back so that he can't move them (see page 48).

If he gets angry and seems to fight against you, make sure that you are not pushing his head towards your breast, instead gently push his shoulders towards you. Also check your 'nose to nipple' position.

Your baby doesn't latch on

Although breastfeeding is natural, it actually takes considerable skill to help your baby attach himself securely to your nipple. Once he's achieved this, he'll take long, peaceful gulps and probably fall asleep at the breast, 'drunk' on milk. It can be extremely upsetting if you can't get your baby latched on to your breast. He'll end up thrashing about, turning his head wildly searching for milk and getting hungrier and more frustrated by the minute.

With a bit of practice, all babies can be taught to latch on (see box, below) and after a few weeks, you'll be popping him under your T-shirt and he'll be sucking within seconds.

In the meantime, be prepared for it to seem a bit fiddly, and also for your baby to 'forget' how to latch on from one feed to the next.

STEP BY STEP TO LATCHING ON

1. Cradle your baby on your lap – this gives you the most control while you get the hang of breastfeeding. Have a pillow behind your lower back because the more comfortable you are, the more relaxed you'll be. Use another pillow on your lap for your baby to lie on – while he's very small this helps get him level with your breast.

2. Adjust your baby so that he's in the tried and tested, 'tummy to mummy, nose to nipple' position (his tummy actually touching you with his nose in line with your nipple). This may feel awkward at first, but getting your baby to lie snugly against you means that he won't have to strain to feed.

3. Gently lift your breast towards your baby's mouth and tickle his chin with your nipple until he opens his mouth really wide, then quickly pop your nipple into his mouth. If he keeps his mouth open wide, and his bottom lip is sticking out around your nipple then he is latched on correctly. But if his mouth or lips look pinched, you'll need to start again because he didn't open his mouth wide enough.

Learning to breastfeed

The easiest way to learn is to have someone with you for each feed showing you exactly what to do. This isn't possible on a busy maternity ward, but do try to get as much help in the hospital as you can, even if you have to keep asking busy nurses to show you what to do.

It's all very well being told by nurses to use the 'tummy to mummy, nose to nipple' technique (see box on page 13) to position your baby correctly, but when you get home from hospital you may find that this all goes out the window and that your baby doesn't seem to be latching on. There is, however, still plenty of help available. Your midwife will visit the day after you get home from hospital and help with feeding, as well as provide details of local breastfeeding support groups; you can also get details of these from your GP. Your midwife should have a 24-hour number, or you could try calling a breastfeeding helpline such as the National Childbirth Trust (NCT) and La Leche League UK (see page 289), which are available 24 hours.

If, after a few days, you're really struggling to breastfeed your baby, you could seek help from a specialist breastfeeding counsellor, usually based at big hospitals. These women are specifically trained to solve breastfeeding problems.

How to tell if you are breastfeeding correctly

There's no way of 'measuring' how much breast milk your baby is getting, but if he's gaining weight, seems happy and sleepy after a feed, and has at least eight wet nappies a day, then he's almost certainly feeding well and getting enough milk. You can tell that your baby is latched on and sucking correctly because his mouth will be open wide with his bottom lip sticking out, you'll see his jaw muscles working, and you'll hear him swallowing. If his lips are pinched into a 'kissing' shape, his cheeks are sucked in and he makes clicking noises, then he's probably not latched on so won't be getting enough milk.

What to do if you can't breastfeed your baby

Should you find yourself unable to feed a desperately hungry baby in the middle of the night with no one to help you until the morning, then express some milk into a small receptacle or cup that your baby can sip from. The hospital has purpose-made ones, so ask to take a few home. Or failing that, the plastic teat cover of a baby bottle works well. Make sure it is sterilised, or at least soaked in boiling water for 45 minutes. If you don't have a breast pump, express by hand straight into the cup simply by squeezing each breast. Then sit your baby up and let him sip from the cup. He'll probably lap it like a cat. A lot will get spilt and if you're short of milk (highly likely if you're stressed and tired) you could always use formula.

Breastfeeding experts advise against using a bottle in the early stages because the baby will get confused switching from a plastic teat to his mother's nipple, and the sucking technique is different. But others will quietly tell you that babies are actually very good at adapting, and that if you're desperate, a bottle is okay in emergencies and won't affect breastfeeding. Keep offering your baby your breast as this increases milk production.

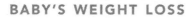

BABY'S WEIGHT LOSS

It's normal for a baby to lose up to 10 per cent of his birth weight in the first 10 days before starting to gain weight, especially if he is breasfed. This is partly because he's not very good at feeding yet, but also because his kidneys haven't matured so produce large volumes of very dilute urine. If your baby is full term this isn't a problem because he'll have enough fat and fluid to carry him through. Premature babies will almost certainly be kept in hospital until they have started gaining weight.

Bottle-feeding

A big drawback of bottle-feeding is the disapproval you'll get from the die-hard 'breast is best' brigade. But there's now a backlash against those who criticise mothers for bottle-feeding. This is because midwives are realising that most women would rather breastfeed but end up bottle-feeding because they struggle so much.

So if breastfeeding hasn't worked for you, or you've simply decided to bottle-feed from the start, don't waste time and energy feeling guilty. You are in the majority as most British women bottle-feed at some stage, and babies thrive on bottled milk. You may also opt for 'mixed' feeding – using a combination of breast and bottled milk (see page 53).

Mothers used to make up six bottles at a time then refrigerate them to be used later. But now safety advice says that ideally you should make up each bottle as you need it to minimise the risk of your baby getting an infection from the powdered milk (powdered milk isn't sterile). Realistically you probably won't stick to this rather stringent safety advice at night, but any paediatric ward nurse will tell you that it is fine to make up several bottles at bedtime and keep them in the fridge overnight. Just ensure that you don't keep made-up milk longer than 24 hours, and if your baby only wants a few sips, you must throw the rest away. You'll waste a lot of milk this week and get through more than six bottles in 24 hours, but this is normal and won't continue. Let your baby have as many feeds as he wants this week.

Once milk comes out of the fridge, be it bottled or breast, it can't be put back in the fridge later and must be thrown away.

HOW TO STOP YOUR BREASTS PRODUCING MILK (AND DEAL WITH BREAST ENGORGEMENT)

If you've decided not to breastfeed, you will need to stop your milk production. Don't express it as this stimulates your milk. Remove just enough milk (by hand) to make yourself more comfortable. You can also put cabbage leaves in your bra – these fit around your breasts, are cooling and soothing, and are thought to reduce milk flow. Studies have found that cabbage leaves are one of the most effective ways to treat engorged breasts. Although no one knows exactly why, one theory is that sulphur in the leaves acts as an anti-irritant and helps relieve inflammation. Icepacks and bags of frozen peas can also give some relief. And you can try taking ibuprofen – anti-inflammatory painkillers are the most effective for breast engorgement.

Note: Paracetamol is the safest painkiller if you are breastfeeding. Breastfeeding mums can also take ibuprofen, but should never take aspirin, which is contraindicated in all children under 12 years because it can cause a liver toxicity disorder known as Reyes Syndrome.

NAPPIES

Number of wet nappies over 24 hours: 8–12
Number of dirty nappies over 24 hours: 0–12

In this first week, you probably won't have much idea how often you should change your baby's nappy. As a guide, change him about every three hours – less often at night. You'll also be concerned about what's a 'normal' nappy. If your baby has fewer than six wet nappies in 24 hours it can indicate dehydration, as can dark, yellow urine. Urine should be almost colourless, and nappies should be heavy. More than eight wet nappies a day show that your baby is getting plenty of fluid.

For the first few days, bowel movements are composed of meconium – sticky, thick, black-green stools with very little smell. This is made of digested mucus and collects in the bowel while your baby is in the womb. As your baby takes milk, his bowel movements will gradually change to a brown-yellow colour and may become 'explosive'. This takes another few days. If you're breastfeeding then your baby's bowel movements will be light yellow and runny, looking much like French mustard. If you're bottle-feeding they will be more solid and browner.

As the milk bowel movements become established, your baby may have a dirty nappy after every feed and you'll probably be changing a lot of nappies towards the end of the week. You can always peep in his leg-hole to see if he's dirty and needs changing, instead of undressing him.

WASHING

You don't have to bath your baby this week, although you might like to if your midwife is around to show you how. But you should 'top and tail' him every day, which means washing his face and bottom. Use cotton wool and warm water (boiled and cooled is best but tap water is okay) and use separate bowls for his bottom and face. You can also use cotton wool to dry him, but you don't need any soap or shampoo. Use 100 per cent cotton wool, which is more absorbent than mixed fibre. Begin by wiping each eye with a separate piece of wet cotton wool, then clean the rest of his face – babies get milk and sick under their chins and behind their ears (don't wash inside the ears though).

You can also clean your baby's scalp – he'll probably have so little hair that you can dry him off in seconds using more cotton wool balls. And if your baby has a lot of hair, use a hairdryer on a cool and low setting – he'll probably enjoy it. Make sure his face is dry before you wash his bottom so that he doesn't feel cold. When washing your baby's bottom, begin by using the old nappy to wipe away any poo, then clean around his bottom and creases with wet cotton wool balls. Once again, dry him with cotton wool. It's better to resist using baby wipes at this stage, even though they are extremely convenient. Even the fragrance-free ones contain chemicals and your baby is still very young.

Wipe a baby boy's testicles and penis, but don't pull back the foreskin. Wipe a baby girl from front to back so that you don't transfer bacteria from her bowels to her bladder. Wipe her genitals, but don't pull open the labia to clean inside.

Cord stump

Newborns are usually sent home from hospital with a plastic clamp on their belly buttons, which seals off the umbilical cord. The newly tied cord can look quite raw, and it may be a bit moist – this is normal. After a few days the stump dries up and turns black, then will drop off between one and four weeks, revealing a brand new belly button.

In the meantime, fold the front of the nappy down to stop it rubbing the cord. You should also check the smell of the cord stump – mildly unpleasant is normal, but if the stump starts to smell really unpleasant, this could indicate an infection, especially if it oozes, or if the surrounding skin becomes red and hot. See your GP straight away if this happens.

You can bath your baby before the cord stump drops off, but dry the cord carefully afterwards with clean tissues and cotton wool. Keep the stump clean by gently dabbing it every other day or so with cotton wool and water, and dry it carefully, again with clean cotton wool. Although the stump looks very sensitive, touching it won't hurt your baby.

When the stump eventually drops off, there may be slight bleeding and it can take a couple of weeks for the new belly button to dry out completely. If it remains moist and smelly for longer than this, mention it to your GP or midwife.

DEVELOPMENT AND PLAYING

Your baby can see up to a distance of 30 cm/12 in, and although his vision is blurred, he can watch your face. He'll be more responsive to faces than anything else this week. The eye's retina cells aren't yet fully developed, so colours look muted to your baby; a black-and-white mobile above the changing table or his cot is about the only 'toy' that a newborn will notice.

Your baby will be familiar with your voice from when he was in the womb, and will quickly get to know your smell so will feel more comforted in your arms than in other people's. If you touch your baby's palm, he'll grasp your finger. He'll also curl his toes when you touch the sole of his foot. These are primitive reflexes that babies are born with. Other newborn reflexes include the rooting reflex. Stroke your baby's cheek and he'll turn towards your finger thinking it's a breast. Babies are also born knowing how to swallow, and they have a natural sucking reflex – put a (clean) finger gently in his mouth and you'll be surprised by the strength of his suck.

!SAFETY TIP OF THE WEEK!
Get a car seat

Hospitals won't let you take your baby home by car without a proper car seat, so make sure you've got one and that you know how to fit it. Newborn seats are designed to be fitted facing the back of the car. The safest place for a child seat is in the rear of the car. If you fit your child seat in the front, make sure any airbag is switched off or decommissioned by a garage. If an airbag went off in a crash it could kill your baby so if you can't switch it off, don't put the baby in the front seat.

Most baby car seats work using existing car seat belts, which can leave some movement even when the seat is properly fitted. But another system available in many newer cars, called Isofix, is considered superior and safer as it attaches directly to the car's frame, eliminating any slack. Whichever seat you buy, it's essential you know how to use it in order for it to offer proper protection to your baby.

WHEN TO SEE A DOCTOR

Jaundice

This condition occurs when a baby's immature liver cannot get rid of the overload of red blood cells that were needed while in the womb. Jaundice develops at about 24 hours after birth, peaks on about day three and usually fades within 10 days. Look out for the whites of your baby's eyes and his skin turning yellow. Neonatal jaundice is rarely a problem and affects 60 per cent of babies.

If jaundice persists beyond a couple of weeks, your midwife may suggest a blood test and treatment. Your baby will have phototherapy for severe jaundice, which involves sleeping under an ultraviolet light. These light waves are absorbed by his skin to help eliminate the overload of red blood cells. Putting your baby by a sunny window can also help to treat jaundice, but take care because your baby may become too hot if he's left too long in his sunny spot. It also helps to feed him frequently – every two to three hours.

Dehydration

Some breastfed babies can become dehydrated during the first week if a new mum doesn't realise that her baby isn't feeding properly. This may be because he isn't latching on (see page 12), or simply isn't feeding often enough.

Signs of dehydration include dry nappies, and the soft non-bony area on his head, the fontanelle, being sunken. As dehydration becomes more severe, your baby may be listless and too tired to feed, his lips will become dry, and he'll lose more than 10 per cent of his birth weight.

If you're worried about dehydration, speak to your midwife urgently because a lack of fluid and salts can make your baby extremely ill. Although severe dehydration is rare, it needs urgent hospital treatment; your baby may be put on a drip or have a feeding tube inserted into his tummy via his nose. To prevent dehydration, make sure your baby is latched on correctly (see page 12). Also, be aware that some babies are very docile in the first week, so if your baby isn't 'demanding' food, then feed him every three hours during the day, and every four hours at night.

WHAT'S HAPPENING TO MUM

Bleeding after the birth is normal, it will be like a very heavy period – use sanitary pads, not tampons, to minimise your risk of infection.

If you pass a clot larger than a 50 pence piece speak to your midwife as you could have some of the placenta still inside you.

Baby blues affects up to 80 per cent of women, so be prepared to feel quite tearful on about day five. This usually disappears quickly as fluctuating hormones settle down. Exhaustion can make the baby blues seem worse so try to get more sleep. This isn't easy because you've got a new baby to look after, but even if you just manage a nap during the day it will make a big difference.

A temperature higher than 38°C/100.4°F could indicate an infection, although some women get a fever and feel shivery when their milk comes in after about three days. If you have a high temperature, speak to your midwife to rule out any problems.

When your milk comes in, usually between days three and five, your breasts may become engorged with milk. This is relieved by frequent feeding. Hot flannels and warm baths can also help get the milk flowing and soften the breasts.

You may also experience painful 'let down' – this is when your milk is released ready for a feed and is often triggered by your baby crying. For some women this can feel like a sharp, burning sensation in the breasts, but it is over in seconds and by about week five will no longer occur.

If you had a Caesarean, there may be a small amount of fluid oozing from the incision, which is blood and other fluids that have accumulated under the incision. This is nothing to worry about, but if oozing persists for longer than a day, tell your midwife as sometimes the incision can open.

If you had an episiotomy (a surgical cut to enlarge the vagina for delivery) or tear, it will probably still be sore this week so you'll need to take painkillers. Paracetamol is safe to take while breastfeeding. If you need something stronger, try paracetamol with codeine (also safe) although it can cause constipation. Sitting on bags of frozen peas can be soothing, or try a rubber ring, made for women who have just given birth and available from large pharmacists. Avoid having salt baths as this can shrink your stitches.

Piles can also make you very sore and many women find that the strain of delivery enlarges any pregnancy piles they may already have. The good news is that even the big piles will probably disappear by themselves over the next couple of months. But in the meantime, avoid constipation or standing up for too long – both of these can make piles worse. And speak to your pharmacist about creams that can help reduce swelling and pain. Sometimes, stitches can stop the blood draining freely which can add to your discomfort – try doing pelvic floor exercises and tightening your anus to encourage blood flow. And do seek further help from your doctor if you are really uncomfortable.

You may get cramps while breastfeeding because hormones stimulate your womb to contract back to its normal size. Again you can take paracetamol.

Passing urine will probably sting for a couple of days. Try pouring warm water over yourself as you wee, or you could try weeing while sitting in a warm bath. If the discomfort goes on for more than several days, speak to your midwife to eliminate a urinary infection. Your first bowel movement after giving birth will be stressful, especially if you've had stitches. But the best advice is to just get on with it, it's never as bad as you think and you won't burst your stitches. If you've not been to the toilet four days after giving birth then drink masses of water and take prune juice.

Don't worry if you didn't bond with your baby the moment you saw him – it's more common for mums to bond in the first week than on first sight, and nearly one in 10 bond some time after the first week. So if it hasn't happened yet, it will. Sometimes mums find it difficult to bond with their babies because they are suffering from post-natal depression (see page 93). Speak to your GP or midwife if, after two weeks, you still feel as though you are struggling to bond.

If you tried breastfeeding and it didn't work out then take heart in the fact that feeding your baby for just one day would have given his immunity a boost and helped protect him from infection.

PLANNING AHEAD
Order a breast pump

If you're breastfeeding and wish to express your milk, order a breast pump. You can buy an electric pump (try the Medela one, www.medela. com), hire one from the NCT or buy a hand pump from your pharmacist – the Avent is popular with a lot of mums. Allow a few days for delivery, and also allow for your pharmacist not having one in stock, in which case you'll need to order one.

There are advantages to both types: electric pumps are much quicker to use, but hand pumps are portable and therefore ideal for sneaking into the office if you return to work while still breastfeeding.

You don't need to express milk this week, apart from by hand in emergencies when your baby won't suck properly (see page 14). Generally speaking, it's better to avoid expressing too early because your baby is still learning to latch on, and expressing can mean giving him a bottle, which requires a different sucking technique. That's why we recommend using a cup to feed him in an emergency.

Ultimately, expressing milk will give you the freedom to go out for longer periods without your baby. And, in the meantime, a breast pump can be used to help stimulate your milk – this may be useful in the early weeks if you are short of milk for some reason.

week 1

The flurry of your hospital homecoming is over and it's time to embark on your first week alone with your baby, who is already a week old. By now your mum has probably packed her bags and gone home, the midwife will pay her last visit this week, and your partner may well be back at work. Gradually you're being left on your own, which can be both exciting and daunting.

Be reassured that there is still plenty of support out there. Your health visitor will be in touch this week and your GP won't give you or your baby the all-clear until week six. In the meantime, don't hesitate to raise any concerns with your health visitor or GP, who will be more than happy to offer reassurance or perhaps a referral to a specialist if they think it necessary.

This week you will probably venture out of the house for the first time with your baby, although just getting out of the front door can be a challenge in itself – it's normal to take two hours or more to get ready in the early weeks. The following tips may help reduce this time, but a lot of it is down to your baby's temperament and bowel movements. Try leaving almost immediately after a feed as this will mean that your baby won't cry from hunger for a good hour or so; change your baby's nappy before the feed and put a bib on him, so that if he's sick you won't have to change his clothes; have a nappy bag already packed, together with everything you need, such as your keys and your mobile phone.

So far it sounds quite straightforward, but what will probably happen is that your baby will need another nappy change after his feed and then wee while you're changing him. Then, by the time you've put him in fresh clothes, he'll be hungry again.

Your only option in this case is to start the nappy and feed cycle again and hope for better luck the second time round. There's no point in leaving the house with a hungry baby as he'll scream and you'll end up turning back within 10 minutes.

SLEEP

Total sleep required: 16–20 hours a day
Pattern: irregular

It's still too soon for your baby to have grasped the concept of day and night, so brace yourself for another tough week of broken sleep. Although it seems that this intense stage of getting no sleep will never end, you'll notice that towards the end of the week your baby will sleep for slightly longer before waking for a feed.

All babies develop their day and night rhythms within a few weeks, but you can speed things along by trying the following. At night, keep the lights low during feeds (just use a bedside light), don't smile or talk, and avoid eye contact. Don't worry about being 'unfriendly', your baby will be comforted by your smell and touch, and of course the milk that you give him.

To teach him about daytime, don't let him sleep for longer than three hours at a time during the day, and don't try to keep ambient noise levels down – for example feel free to use the television, washing machine and the phone. It's useful if your baby learns to sleep through noise because it means that when he's older, you won't have to tiptoe around.

Cot death

Like most mothers, you will probably worry about cot death, particularly in the early weeks when your baby looks so tiny and vulnerable. And feeling exhausted can make the anxiety worse. But cot death, or Sudden Unexplained Death in Infancy (SUDI), is rare – it affects just 300 babies in the UK per year – that's less than one in 2,000. It peaks in months two and three, then drops off quickly and hardly ever occurs after six months.

Although the cause of cot death isn't known, the latest thinking is that it may be caused by an undetected defect in the heart rhythm. Another theory is that the part of the brain that tells us when we can't breathe properly is underdeveloped which means that the baby doesn't wake up if he's having breathing problems.

There's plenty you can do to minimise your baby's risk, and once you've taken these precautions there's little point in worrying too much. If you find that you're constantly anxious and checking your baby's breathing more than once or twice a night, speak to your midwife or GP as they will be able to reassure you.

Reducing the risk of cot death

Put your baby to sleep on his back

This is the safest sleeping position and cot death has dropped in the UK by 75 per cent since a 'Back to Sleep' campaign was introduced in 1991 to put babies to sleep on their backs. Being on his back won't make your baby more likely to choke if he possets some milk as he will automatically turn his head to the side – vomiting is not a cause of cot death. You may discover that your baby seems more comfortable on his tummy and is easier to settle – don't let him get into this habit as it's safer for him to sleep on his back, even for short naps during the day. And don't let him sleep on his side as he may easily roll on to his front.

Don't smoke

Now that nearly all babies sleep on their backs, smoking is the biggest risk factor affecting cot death. Don't let anyone smoke in your home and keep your baby away from cigarette smoke. If you or your partner smoke, only do so outside, keep smoky clothes out of the bedroom, and never let your baby sleep in your bed as this has been shown to increase the risk of cot death.

Breastfeed

Studies have shown that the risk of cot death is three times lower for breastfed babies compared with bottle-fed babies. No one knows the reason for this, but one theory is that there is more awareness between the mother and baby.

Keep your baby cool

Overheating is a known factor in cot death so don't bundle your baby up in too many clothes and blankets, and never put a hat on him when he is sleeping indoors – he needs to lose heat from his head. Ideally, try to keep the bedroom at around 16–20°C/61–68°F – warm enough to feel comfortable in your nightwear with a dressing gown on. There's no need to panic when the temperature soars in summer because cot death is actually more likely to occur in the winter months – this is thought to be because people wrap their babies up too much.

As a general rule, your baby should wear one more layer than you to feel comfortable. For a more specific guide as to what your baby should wear in bed, see the blanket guide box (overleaf).

BLANKET GUIDE
WHAT YOUR BABY SHOULD WEAR IN BED

Above 26°C/79°F – no blankets, your baby should wear a vest only.

24–26°C/75–79°F – no blankets, your baby should wear a sleepsuit.

21–24°C/70–75°F – one blanket, your baby should wear a vest only/or no blankets, your baby should wear a vest and sleepsuit.

18–21°C/64.5–70°F – one blanket, your baby should wear a sleepsuit.

16–18°C/61–64.5°F – two blankets, your baby should wear a vest and a sleepsuit.

Below 16°C/61°F – three blankets, your baby should wear a vest and a sleepsuit.

Make your baby's bed safe

Always put your baby in the 'feet to foot' position in his cot or Moses basket. This means that his feet are near the foot of his bed – the idea is that as he wriggles, he moves up his bed away from the bedding and his head doesn't get covered by the bedding.

Don't use cot bumpers, duvets or pillows as there's a small chance these can suffocate babies. A cellular blanket (the cotton ones with holes in them specifically designed for babies) works well – tuck it around the mattress and only let it go as high as your baby's chest, don't tuck him in up to his chin.

Another good bedding option is a baby sleeping bag – these can be expensive as you need bigger sizes as your baby grows, but lots of mums say it's worth it because their babies sleep better because they feel wrapped up and secure.

Keep your baby's Moses basket or cot in your room for the first six months and try to avoid letting your baby have his daytime naps in a separate room for at least the first three months. This has been shown to reduce the risk of cot death. Avoid using a second-hand or borrowed mattress. Nearly half of all babies who die of cot death have raised levels of a toxin produced by *Staphylococcus aureus* bacteria, which thrive in damp foam. Most mattresses nowadays are waterproof and have plastic covers to reduce the risk.

CRYING

Number of hours your baby may cry in a day: 2–4 is usual, but some babies can cry for up to 12 hours

It's normal for your baby to cry a bit more this week and this will continue until about week six when his crying will probably peak. Crying is your baby's way of communicating, although in the early weeks this can be pretty stressful as you'll only be able to make random guesses as to what he needs. His number one request is still for food, so always try offering him milk.

Excessive crying

If your baby is going to be an excessive crier, then this is probably the week that he will show his true colours. A perfectly healthy baby can cry for up to 12 hours, pretty much non-stop. Of course you can try feeding, burping, rocking and nappy changing – but if nothing works you will end up feeling disheartened and very concerned about your baby. In this case it's advisable to see your GP or midwife because they will be able to eliminate any medical problems. Knowing that your baby is okay will make you feel less anxious and this in itself may reduce your baby's crying.

Relatives and friends with baby experience are invaluable at this time as they can relieve you of your screaming infant. Just try not to feel like a bad mother when your baby stops crying the instant someone else takes him – remember that they are less emotionally involved and sleep deprived than you.

Sometimes mothers are admitted to hospital with their crying newborns – not because there's anything physically wrong with the baby, but simply to give mum a break and a chance to get some sleep and regain her sanity when she's at her absolute wits' end.

FEEDING

Total milk required: 540–690 ml/18–23 oz a day
(up to 90 ml/3 oz per feed)
Pattern: irregular, up to 12 feeds a day

Your baby is very new to feeding, so don't be surprised if he still seems a little confused at times. Whether he's drinking from a bottle or breastfeeding, it requires a knack for him to position the teat or nipple in his mouth correctly and he may forget what to do from one feed to the next. So the best thing you can do this week is to keep practising and not expect too much. You should still be demand feeding and not worrying about routines. You'll find that sometimes your baby may go for four hours between feeds, but at other times he'll want a top-up after just an hour.

Breastfeeding

A lot of women give up breastfeeding around now because of difficulties such as insufficient milk and sore nipples. It can be incredibly stressful when you've got a hungry, screaming newborn demanding milk. But persevere because once you've cracked breastfeeding, you'll find it effortless, and much more convenient than using a bottle as you can feed your baby instantly and anywhere. And, of course, your baby will reap the benefits of breast milk (see page 11).

Why you may want to give up breastfeeding this week

Sore, cracked nipples

If you're kicking your feet in agony every time you feed your baby, you're certainly not alone – cracked, blistered and bleeding nipples are extremely common in the early stages. Understandably a lot of women give up because of this, but there are steps you can take to help you through the next few days while you heal.

The most likely cause of sore nipples is your baby not latching on properly (see page 12), so make sure that his lips cover the areola and that his mouth is open wide. When you are learning to breastfeed, you'll probably feel so relieved that your baby is sucking at all that you won't want to interrupt his feed. But if it feels uncomfortable then stop immediately because you can get a blister after just 15 minutes. To stop your baby mid-feed, slide your finger into his mouth to break the suction with your breast.

When you latch him on correctly, you should feel less pain. But correct latching on won't bring much relief if your nipples are already sore and cracked. If this is the case, then the bad news is that you need to keep breastfeeding through the pain, otherwise your milk will dry up – in desperate cases you can give your baby expressed milk for a couple of days. But the sooner you get back to letting your baby suckle the better because breastfeeding does actually 'toughen up' your nipples as well as elongate flatter nipples. So perseverance will result in longer, tougher nipples that won't require quite such precise latching-on techniques.

Try not to be put off because when you get through this discomfort, feeding your baby will actually feel quite nice. In the meantime, you may like to try using a cream. Lansinoh for Breastfeeding Mothers is probably the most effective nipple cream and is endorsed by La Leche League UK (see page 289). It isn't available from all chemists, so be prepared to shop around. Made from lanolin, it forms a thick sticky barrier over the nipple to take the edge off the pain of feeding, and it is soothing to apply after a feed. You can also take a paracetamol with codeine painkiller 15 minutes before a feed – this is powerful but won't harm your baby while you're breastfeeding. Be aware that codeine can cause constipation after a couple of days. And also if the maximum dose is taken for more than three weeks, some people can get addicted.

As a last resort you can try nipple shields. These will make feeding instantly less painful but your baby won't get as much milk because shields have been shown to reduce milk production. Another drawback is that your baby may become used to sucking a shield and find it difficult to go back to sucking directly from the nipple. But if it's a matter of using shields or giving up on breastfeeding, it's certainly worth giving them a go – limit them to every other feed if you can, or just use them on your more painful nipple. Flatter nipples are more prone to soreness, but your baby will gradually draw them out. Wearing nipple shields slows down the elongation of nipples – another reason to try to avoid them.

Insufficient milk

Sometimes women think they're not producing enough milk when in fact there isn't a problem. If your baby is gaining weight and has plenty of wet and dirty nappies then don't worry as you've obviously got enough and there is no need to try to 'measure' your milk by expressing.

But if you're still concerned, and your baby becomes fretful rather than soothed by a feed, try expressing after the feed. If you find that you are unable to express more than half an ounce from both breasts within 10 minutes, then you're short of milk and can take the following steps to boost your production:

- Firstly, continue to express after every daytime feed – do this for a week and you'll notice that you quickly produce more milk. You can throw this milk away as there won't be much initially and you want your baby to be hungry and do lots of sucking at the next feed. You could give the expressed milk to your baby if he isn't gaining weight quickly enough – seek advice from your midwife or health visitor.

- Make sure that you are feeding on demand, letting your baby take as long as he wants, and offering him both breasts. The more your breasts are stimulated, the more milk they produce.
- Ensure that you don't become dehydrated as this reduces milk production – have at least three litres of water a day and drink throughout the night – have a jug of water in the bedroom.
- Don't smoke because this has been shown to reduce milk production. Smoking also affects your 'let down' reflex, which triggers the flow of milk at feeding times or when your baby cries.
- It's also thought that avoiding stress, eating regularly and having warm baths and showers increases milk production. So have a few lazy sessions with your baby just lying with him on the bed, letting him feed whenever he wants while you drink plenty of water, eat what you like, read magazines or watch TV. Doing this each day will force you to stop trying to do the housework and will definitely help milk production.

DON'T RUSH YOUR BABY'S FEEDS

If your baby seems to want to take his time and sucks very sporadically towards the end of the feed it means that he's drunk what's known as the 'fore' milk, which is thirst quenching, and has now reached the 'hind' milk, which is richer and more filling. So don't be in a hurry to end the feeding session or to switch breasts when he seems to have slowed his pace.

Bottle-feeding

Your baby should be much better at feeding from a bottle this week and be taking 60–90 ml/2–3 oz per feed. It's still too early for a feeding routine, so continue to follow your baby's demands and be prepared for another week of throwing away lots of un-drunk milk.

Cleaning the bottles

Once you get organised, bottle-feeding will seem almost effortless. The only potentially serious problem is not cleaning the bottles properly and infecting your baby with bacteria that could give him diarrhoea. Warm milk is the perfect breeding ground for bacteria and your baby still has a weak immune system.

To minimise the risk, it is essential to clean and sterilise your bottles properly. So immediately after each feed, thoroughly rinse the bottle, teat and cap in warm water – this stops milk drying on to the bottles. When you have a little more time, use a bottle brush and some washing-up liquid and scrub everything in soapy water. Finally, rinse everything thoroughly, then sterilise.

You've probably found that sterilising the bottles is a major part of bottle-feeding and can take quite some time. So make sure that you use a method that suits you because baby bottles need to be sterilised up until six months (after which you can use a dishwasher if you have one). If you don't, then you will have to sterilise for a year.

Sterilising tablets

This is the cheapest way to sterilise, and useful if you are travelling, but it is a bit more fiddly and time consuming than other sterilising methods. You simply add a tablet to four pints of cold water in a large non-metallic container and leave bottles, teats, rings and caps submerged for at least 30 minutes. To make up the bottles for a feed, wash your hands then rinse the bottles and teats with freshly boiled water, fill them with milk immediately, cover the teats with a sterilised cap and place in the fridge.

Steamers

Slightly larger than a kettle, these plastic containers can be plugged in and kept on a kitchen worktop. After washing out the milk bottles, you arrange them in the steamer, add a little water then switch it on. It takes around eight minutes, after which everything is ready to use. Depending on the model, you can steam about six bottles at a time, and a steamer costs around £40.

Microwave steamers

These are similar to electric steamers, but instead of plugging them in you put them in the microwave for five minutes. They are half the size and about half the price (around £20), but you can only steam up to four bottles at a time.

NAPPIES

Number of wet nappies over 24 hours: 8–12
Number of dirty nappies over 24 hours: 0–12

By the end of this week you will have changed over 100 nappies, and may feel that nappies have taken over your life. But this will improve as you get quicker (it will take you less than five minutes to change a nappy by next week), and also as your baby starts to dirty his nappy less frequently.

At the moment, his kidneys are still immature, which means that he produces high volumes of dilute urine. And his immature bowels mean he may have a bowel movement after every feed (or he might only go once every other day – both of these patterns are normal).

The best tip for this week is to keep a roll of kitchen paper next to your changing table. This is because your baby is going to the toilet so frequently at the moment that he's extremely likely to do so during a nappy change. Your baby may have bowel movements throughout the night because his internal body clock has not yet been set. It's exhausting changing nappies in the small hours of the morning, but you don't have to change your baby's nappy at every night feed if he's feeding more than every three hours, has only done a very small poo and hasn't got nappy rash.

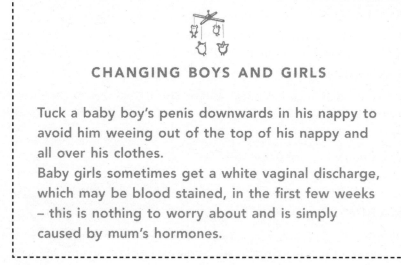

CHANGING BOYS AND GIRLS

Tuck a baby boy's penis downwards in his nappy to avoid him weeing out of the top of his nappy and all over his clothes.

Baby girls sometimes get a white vaginal discharge, which may be blood stained, in the first few weeks – this is nothing to worry about and is simply caused by mum's hormones.

Nappy changing bag

You'll probably venture out of your home with your baby this week and will need to pack up a nappy changing bag. This doesn't have to be big – the key is to keep it topped up so that you're never caught short. Pack it with the following:

- A nappy for every hour that you intend to be out (that's generous but one-week-olds can have a lot of bowel movements in a short space of time).
- A packet of baby wipes – these are more convenient than cotton wool and water and most mums end up switching around now. The downside is that they are more expensive and the smell of the fragranced ones can be a bit overwhelming.
- Something to dry your baby's bottom – an old face cloth works well.

- Nappy bags for dirty nappies.
- A change of clothes in case the nappy leaks.
- A changing mat – you can buy travel mats that fold up small.

WASHING

So far you have been topping and tailing your baby each day, but now you can start bathing him every few days. Bathing your baby for the first time can seem pretty daunting, but you'll quickly get used to it and should feel confident and relaxed after about half a dozen times.

Your baby's first bath

The aim of this first bath isn't to make your baby super clean, but simply to get him used to being in water, and also to give you a bit of practice.

You can use a baby bath, but if you haven't got one the big bath is fine – the only downside is that it can be hard on your back as you lean over to hold your baby. Use a rubber bath mat to stop your baby slipping, or you can buy specially designed plastic baby seats which you attach to the bottom of the bath. Keep the bath shallow, just 5–8 cm/2–3 in deep, as this will make things more manageable.

Make sure the water temperature is not too hot by testing with your wrist or elbow as these are more sensitive to temperature than your hands. Always put the cold water in first to avoid scalding your baby – most burns in young children occur when parents forget to put the cold water into the bath. Be aware, though, that a lot of new mums make the bath water too cold because they're so concerned about scalding their baby. Your baby won't like being plunged into a tepid bath – so make sure it is nice and warm.

Once you've run the bath, undress your baby down to his nappy and wrap him in a towel, then you can pop him on the bathroom floor while you make final temperature adjustments to the water. Remove your baby's nappy, and if he's done a poo you'll need to clean him. Keep his top half covered with the towel while you do this to make him feel warm and secure. Lower your baby slowly into the water, keeping him in a semi-upright position – have one hand around his shoulders and under his armpit, making sure you support his head, and the other under his bottom.

When he is 'sitting' on the bottom of the bath you may be able to remove one hand while still holding him around his shoulders – this gives you a free hand to wash him. What's more likely to happen is that your baby will wriggle, feel incredibly slippery and possibly scream alarmingly, in which case keep holding him with two hands while your partner washes him. You don't have to use shampoo or soap for the first bath – just wash your baby with water using a face cloth (he should have his own). Gently rub the cloth over his face, his hair, under his chin, his armpits, hands and finally his bottom.

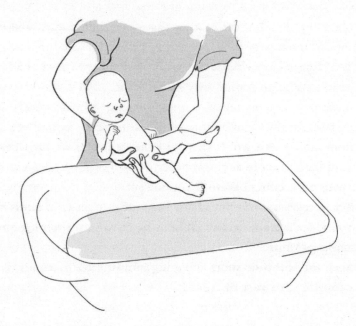

When lowering your baby into the bath, have one hand around his shoulders and under his armpit, and the other under his bottom.

If there's no one around to help and you feel that you need to keep holding your baby with two hands, then just swoosh him in the water for a minute or two and don't even think about washing him.

In the unlikely instance that your baby enjoys his first bath, it's still advisable to take him out after a couple of minutes before he changes his mind and before he gets cold – his inner thermostat is still very underdeveloped and he can't yet control his body temperature very well. So keep the bathroom warm and have a towel ready on the bathroom floor so that you can wrap him up quickly.

What to do if your baby hates his bath

There are a number of reasons why some babies initially hate being bathed, but console yourself that this quickly changes – after you've bathed him about six times he'll probably begin to enjoy it. In the meantime, you may want to think about the following:

- Make sure he's not cold, check the water temperature, and keep the bathroom warm.
- Try keeping him wrapped in a muslin cloth when you bath him as this will help him to feel more secure.
- Bathing your baby when he's tired or hungry will almost certainly result in tears, so pick your moment – about half an hour after a feed works well, and choose a time of day when your baby is more alert, probably in the morning. Don't worry about an evening bathtime routine yet.
- Try to relax because your baby may pick up on your stress if you're feeling anxious about bathing him; keep soothing and smiling at him.
- Keep the bathtime short – dipping him in for 20 seconds is enough if he's very distressed.

DEVELOPMENT AND PLAYING

Your baby will start to recognise your face, and studies show that mothers' faces trigger feelings of pleasure and calm in babies. He'll stare at your face but won't be very good at making eye contact at this stage. Spend a few minutes every day letting him stare at you, perhaps during feeding or nappy changing. Smile and coo at him because he'll find your expressions fascinating.

Continue to touch his palm to trigger his grasp response – this helps develop his finger muscles. Every movement he makes, however tiny, strengthens his muscles. Your baby won't be able to control his head yet – when he's lying down it rests to one side. But when he's in your arms you may notice tiny head movements as he tries to watch your face.

!SAFETY TIP OF THE WEEK!
Put your baby to sleep on his back

Remember to put your baby to sleep on his back. This has been shown to reduce the risk of cot death by 75 per cent. Make sure babysitters and grandparents do the same – older people are more likely to wrongly think it's okay to put a baby to sleep on his front.

WHEN TO SEE A DOCTOR

Noisy breathing

New babies often snuffle and snort, particularly when they're asleep. This can sound alarming, but isn't anything to worry about. They tend to get quite bunged up from spending so much time on their backs and are simply clearing their nasal passages of mucus and debris.

Another likely cause is the common cold, which many babies get in the first few weeks because they're handed around so many friends and relatives. Babies are particularly hard hit by colds for a number of reasons. Firstly, their nasal passages are tiny so they quickly get blocked, and this is made worse by the fact that newborns spend so much time on their backs resulting in mucus pooling in the nasal passages. Another problem is that new babies are obligate nose breathers – this means that they don't learn to breathe through their mouths until they are about six months old. A cold will make your baby cry more than usual and sleep less. Try putting a folded towel under one end of his mattress to tip his head up as this helps excess mucus to drain into his stomach rather than pool in his nasal passages. You can also use ordinary saline nose drops – these aren't specifically for babies and are available over the counter from chemists. Put one or two drops into each nostril before feeds to help clear his passages. Some mums try nasal decongesters, also from chemists, which are designed to clear your baby's nose by inserting a plastic device into the nostril and squeezing a plastic bulb to suck from his nose. But these often don't work very well and babies tend to hate them. An alternative is to actually suck the mucus from your infant's nose and then spit it out – it sounds far worse than it actually is and plenty of brave mums resort to this. You can also buy decongestant drops to put on cot bedding, but these can't be used until your baby is three months old.

Sometimes the common cold can cause more serious problems. Swallowing mucus, for instance, can make babies vomit and lead to dehydration. If your baby throws up a lot of milk feeds then look out for dry nappies – less than four wet nappies a day is worrying.

Because your baby is bunged up, he might find it difficult to suckle which, again, can lead to dehydration. If he's unhappy during a feed – pulling faces, getting angry and crying – it could mean that he's struggling to breathe and feed at the same time and needs help.

Irregular breathing

This is very common and can be worrying for parents, but it's actually normal for a baby to have an irregular breathing pattern and even to pause for breath for up to 10 seconds. This is because the breathing control centre in the brain is still immature.

Occasionally, a baby may stop breathing for longer than 20 seconds – if this happens, take him to your hospital's Emergency Department. Known as an 'apparently life threatening event' (ALTE), this is rare and affects less than 1 per cent of babies. But it should always be assessed in hospital.

A TEMPERATURE ABOVE 38°C/100.4°F

The easiest and most accurate way to take your baby's temperature is with an ear thermometer which will give a reading in seconds. This can indicate an infection, perhaps a chest infection, and should be treated quickly. Don't give your baby Calpol (liquid paracetamol for babies) until he is three months old because although this will bring down his temperature, it will mask any serious problems. But once he has been checked by a doctor your baby can have Calpol from any age.

week 2

Expect a visit from your health visitor this week. She'll be a mine of information about everything from looking after your infant to giving you details of local mother and baby groups. Don't worry about quizzing her – she'll expect you to bombard her with questions and she'll probably have more time than the midwife.

Your health visitor will also tell you about your local baby clinic, where you can go each week to get your baby checked and weighed. And she will give you what's known by everyone as the 'Red Book' – the Personal Child Health Record – if you have not already received it from your midwife. This is a history of your child's growth and development from birth until he's aged 20. Every child in the country has one and, as well as height and weight charts, the Red Book also contains an immunisation record, notes made by the health visitors about your child's progress, plus a record of various milestones such as smiling, getting teeth, crawling, walking and talking that you can fill in. Always take this book along to any health-related appointments your child may have.

You can tear out the growth charts for the opposite sex and keep the book in a plastic bag for protection inside your nappy changing bag so it is always with you.

This week, your health visitor will plot your baby's weight and length in the book. You'll then be able to see from the chart how your two-week-old compares with other babies the same age. There are various lines on the chart called centiles, and if your baby is on the 50th centile it means that he is exactly average. If he's on the 25th centile it means that for every 100 babies, 75 babies plot above him and 25 below him.

You may become anxious if your baby is plotted too far from the 50th centile thinking that your child is too heavy, too light, too tall or too short. But bear in mind that for every 100 children measured, only one will fall on the 50th centile while the rest are spread between the two outermost lines, so it's really not worth worrying about.

SLEEP

Total sleep required: 15–18 hours a day
Pattern: irregular

You'll notice that your baby is more aware of his surroundings this week, which means he doesn't have as much sleep as when he was first born, and also he wakes up more easily – for example if you make a noise or tuck his blankets in. To help him stay asleep for longer, you could try swaddling him – the ancient practice of wrapping a baby snugly in cloth – which has now been proved by scientists to help babies sleep more deeply. This is because it stops their arms jerking about, which can wake them up, and also reminds them of the confined space inside the womb and so makes them feel safe and secure.

Another benefit of swaddling is that it can help to get your baby to sleep in the first place. You'll notice that after a few days of being swaddled, your baby actually recognises being wrapped as a signal that it's time to go to sleep.

Other advantages of swaddling are that it can calm your baby when he's feeling fractious, and also it ensures that he stays on his back, which reduces his risk of cot death – this applies to slightly older babies who are able to turn. Be aware that some babies simply don't like being swaddled, so if yours makes a fuss and seems angry, then give up.

Some babies wriggle out of their swaddling clothes because they weren't swaddled correctly or tightly enough in the first place, or because they've grown more active and are able to kick off their swaddling. This generally happens after week eight, and if it does then it's time to stop swaddling him because a kicked-off blanket can potentially suffocate a baby.

The final swaddling hazard is overheating – so make sure that your baby isn't too warm as this is linked with cot death. NEVER cover his head or face.

How to swaddle your baby

1. Take either a muslin cloth or a cellular blanket (depending on the temperature), and fold the upper corner down.

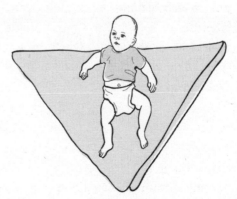

2. Lie your baby on the blanket with his neck in the centre of the fold.

3. Pull the far
   right corner
   of the swaddle
   across over your
   baby's left arm
   and tuck it
   under his right
   buttock. His left
   arm should be
   snugly by his
   side.

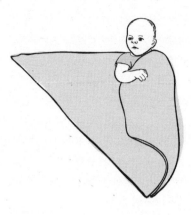

4. Do the same with
   the opposite side of
   the swaddle.

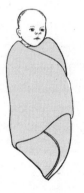

If he sucks his thumb or fingers, usually by week six, then bend one arm so that his fingers peep out of the top of the swaddle near his face.

CRYING

Number of hours your baby may cry in a day: 2–5

Your baby's crying pattern continues to increase and although hunger is still the main cause, he may also cry if he needs to poo, pass wind, burp or even wee. This is thought to be due to a mix-up of sensory messages in the brain which is still too immature to distinguish between pain and other sensations – such as needing to burp.

As a result, your baby translates a lot of the sensory information he receives as discomfort and so cries. Another reason that he gets upset is that he's being bombarded by lots of signals that he doesn't yet understand.

One giveaway sign that he's distressed by wind or needing to poo is that he goes red in the face and grimaces. Pick him up and comfort him and be patient for the next few weeks as his brain gradually learns to distinguish different sensations. Most experts now agree that responding to your baby's crying quickly will result in less crying in the months to come as he will feel more secure. It's no longer thought that parents should let their babies cry it out at this stage.

Providing a womb-like environment for your baby will help him to feel safer and cry less, which is why swaddling can be comforting for babies (see page 48). You might also want to try using a baby carrier or sling. Your baby will be nestled against you and will be lulled to sleep as you move – just like when he was in the womb. He'll be nice and warm and be able to hear you talking and breathing. You can wear a baby carrier when you're out and about with your baby or even as you get on with chores around the house. Studies have shown that babies who are carried in either baby carriers or in their parents' arms for at least three hours a day are more content and cry less in the first 12 weeks. There are lots of slings on the market – all of them are quite complicated to put on so do practise before putting your baby in.

FEEDING

Total milk required: 600–750 ml/20–25 oz a day
(up to 105 ml/3.5 oz per feed)
Pattern: 7–10 feeds a day

You may notice a pattern emerging this week as your baby begins to show the early signs of feeding every three hours. Don't push him too quickly into this pattern as he is very young and still needs to be fed on demand. You probably won't see a clear feeding pattern until about week 12.

A lot of babies go through a growth spurt at around this time, as they are nearly three weeks old. This can last for up to two days and your baby will seem particularly hungry and a bit fractious – especially if you're breastfeeding. You may end up feeding him more often as your milk supply adjusts to his increased demands. But whether you are breast- or bottle-feeding, continue following your baby's demands.

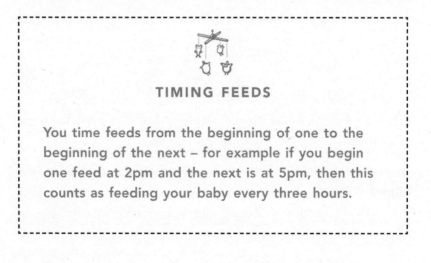

TIMING FEEDS

You time feeds from the beginning of one to the beginning of the next – for example if you begin one feed at 2pm and the next is at 5pm, then this counts as feeding your baby every three hours.

Breastfeeding – supplementing with formula

A lot of mums decide to supplement breastfeeding with a bottle of formula around about now – this generally happens for two reasons. Firstly it could be because your baby has his first growth spurt – if this is the case then you'll find that your baby is suddenly much hungrier and asking for more milk than you are producing. It's better to allow your milk supply to increase to meet his needs rather than give him a bottle, otherwise you could end up giving him more and more formula as he grows rather than letting your milk supply increase. The answer is to feed your baby whenever he asks because the extra stimulation will increase your milk supply within a couple of days. After this, he'll stop demanding food quite so often and will be better tempered.

The other reason why lots of women introduce a bottle at this stage is that they find their milk supply dwindles in the evening when they're tired. Giving your baby formula at this time is a quick-fix way to quieten him and it may also help him to sleep for longer as formula is heavier than breast milk. Lots of women happily breastfeed for months adding an additional bottle of formula in the evenings. But if you want to stick solely to breast milk then try expressing in the morning when you have the most milk and giving it to your baby in the evening. You could also feed your baby more in the evening to help increase your evening milk. Or you could just give your baby an evening bottle in 'emergencies', for example when you're particularly tired and don't have the milk. If you only do this every few days or so, it shouldn't affect your evening supply.

Mixed feeding

By now your baby has probably learnt to 'latch on' (see page 12) and so shouldn't have a problem switching back and forth from breast to bottle. What can happen if you give your baby a bottle before he's learnt to latch on is that he discovers how easy it is to suck milk from a bottle and so decides not to bother with the breast any more, especially if it's been a struggle.

Choosing formula

You will have noticed quite a choice of formula milk in the shops and have probably wondered which is the most suitable for your baby. Discuss this with your health visitor, but generally speaking the best option is one that contains a high proportion of whey as this is closer to breast milk. Most formula milks that are aimed at new babies are high in whey, for example SMA Gold, Farley's First Milk and Aptamil First.

Follow-on milks contain less whey but more casein, which is supposed to satisfy hungry babies after six months – they also contain extra vitamins. Large tins of powdered milk work out to be the most economical, whereas the cartons of made-up milk are very convenient but also more expensive. Avoid alternatives to cows' milk, such as soy or goats' milk formulas, unless your doctor has advised you to use them. These also have allergy and intolerance risks.

NAPPIES

Number of wet nappies over 24 hours: 6–10
Number of dirty nappies over 24 hours: 0–10

Nappy rash

It's quite common for nappy rash to develop about now so watch out for redness around your baby's bottom. The key to treating nappy rash is to act quickly to stop it getting worse – some babies' bottoms become so red and sore that they bleed, and this can take as little as a few hours. But the upside is that a few hours of the correct treatment can greatly reduce the discomfort and make a noticeable improvement as babies' skin heals quicker than adults'.

Cause

Nappy rash is a result of urine being broken down by bacteria in the stools to form ammonia. Ammonia burns the skin causing red, sore and sometimes bleeding skin. Constant pooing at this age can make nappy rash particularly bad, but in a couple of weeks your baby will poo less frequently which will improve things.

Prevention

Change your baby's nappy frequently, and immediately after he has done a poo. Clean him thoroughly using cotton wool and water, or baby wipes designed for sensitive skin as these don't contain alcohol or fragrance. Be meticulous about drying your baby's bottom – a face cloth, cotton wool or even a hairdryer set on cool all work well. Use a barrier cream if your baby is susceptible to nappy rash as this buys you a bit of time between nappy changes and delays ammonia reaching the skin.

Treatment

At the first sign of nappy rash use an antiseptic cream such as Sudocrem or Drapolene – you can use these as a preventative measure for all nappy changes if your baby is very susceptible to severe nappy rash. With nappy cream less is more, so you should only use a thin layer, as a fine film is better than thickly applied cream. Let your baby go without his nappy for as long as possible, just five minutes will help but a couple of hours will be a lot more effective. Keep a clean nappy under his bottom to mop up accidents and let him lie on his changing mat on the floor. For persistent nappy rash, try a titanium-based nappy cream such as Metanium.

WASHING

By now you've probably bathed your baby a few times and are feeling a little more confident. You may well be eager to try out some of the delicious smelling baby bath products available, but it's best to keep things simple as your baby is still very young. Try using a baby shampoo for his hair, bottom and under his chin – you can use this for every other bath to avoid drying his skin.

After the bath you can massage his skin with olive oil or grapeseed oil – both available from chemists. Your baby's skin shouldn't be dry as he's still very young so you won't need to use a moisturiser or body lotion yet, but it can be quite nice to give your baby a gentle massage to help you bond and also to relax him. Try doing clockwise circles on his tummy or soft sweeping strokes on his arms or legs. Keep him covered with a towel so that he doesn't get cold, and play it very much by ear – your baby will let you know what he likes and doesn't, and when he's had enough.

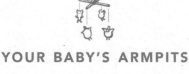

YOUR BABY'S ARMPITS

Don't forget to wash and dry your baby's armpits. He'll probably clamp his arms down during bathtime, which makes washing and drying difficult – lots of new mums discover a cheesy smell after a few weeks if the armpits have not been properly cleaned.

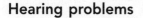

Baby acne

Up to 40 per cent of new babies develop acne about now, thought to be caused by their mothers' hormones still in their systems. Apart from looking unattractive in photos, this isn't a problem and won't bother your baby in the slightest. It will clear up by about week 12, and in the meantime simply wash his face with cotton wool and water and pat dry. Don't apply any lotions or squeeze his spots – he won't have a single scar or blemish if you don't tamper with his skin.

DEVELOPMENT AND PLAYING

Your baby will suddenly look taller as he begins to uncurl from the foetal position and loses his newborn appearance. But his legs will still be bent.

This week your baby will make noises that sound like a cross between crying and shouting. This is the first stage of language development and your baby is practising his vowel sounds.

Your baby may be soothed by 'white noise', for example the car or hairdryer. This is because these sound similar to the muffled noises he heard while he was in the womb. Everything will sound clearer to your baby now there's not a barrier of water in the way.

WHEN TO SEE A DOCTOR

Hearing problems

Every year, around 900 babies in the UK are born deaf or with a hearing impairment. The earlier a baby's hearing problem is picked up, the fewer problems he will have with speech, social and emotional development. So it's important to ensure your baby is tested.

Has your baby been screened?

Ideally your baby will have either been screened in hospital before discharge, or by your health visitor some time this week. But because the screening programme is still being implemented, there's a chance that your baby hasn't been tested – in which case ask your GP or health visitor to be put in touch with your local screening service.

How the hearing test works

It's quick and painless and involves putting an earpiece into your baby's ear and playing soft clicking sounds. If your baby can hear, the cochlea in his inner ear will produce sounds in response to the clicks, which are recorded on a computer. The test takes a few minutes and is often done while your baby is sleeping.

The results

If your baby has a problem he will have further tests and he may be fitted with a hearing aid. You will be given lots of information and support on how to help your baby. But even if your baby is given the all-clear, you should still observe his hearing in everyday life as some problems develop later. Do loud noises make him startle, and as he gets older, does he turn towards sounds such as your voice? Glue ear can be a cause of hearing loss (see page 258).

> ## !SAFETY TIP OF THE WEEK!
> ### Don't shake your baby
>
> If your baby won't stop crying and won't go to sleep, it can push the patience of even the most experienced mother. If you find yourself wanting to shake your baby to make him quiet, you certainly won't be alone. Nearly all mums get desperate at some stage, but

thankfully very few actually lose control – just a few shakes could be enough to cause brain damage or even kill a baby. If you find yourself at your wits' end, hand your baby to your partner or anyone else who's around – or failing that simply put him safely in his cot, close the door and walk away. You'll be surprised how quickly you calm down and how your baby once again becomes the cutest little thing in the world (even though he's still screaming almost continuously). If you do ever lose control and shake your baby, seek immediate medical help. Even if your baby seems fine, there could be bleeding in the brain which may need medical or surgical treatment. For more help with crying babies call the charity Cry-sis helpline on 08451 228 669, open seven days a week from 9am until 10pm. They will put you in touch with a volunteer in your area who is also a parent and has been through similar problems.

WHAT'S HAPPENING TO MUM

If you are still bleeding this week, it will be much lighter. Speak to your GP if this isn't the case.

Lots of women find that they are anaemic after giving birth, particularly if they had a Caesarean. Signs to look out for are extreme tiredness and your lower inside eyelids being pale instead of a rich pink colour. Talk to your pharmacist about taking an iron supplement, or an iron-rich tonic.

You may have some pelvic pain because the spaces between the joints expanded during pregnancy and birth. If this hasn't eased and is bothering you, then speak to your GP or midwife who can refer you to a physiotherapist.

If you're breastfeeding, you may get a blocked milk duct – a hard red patch on your breast. Check that your bra isn't too tight, and make sure that your baby drains the blocked breast completely before swapping him over. Hot baths, hot flannels and massaging the sore spot can help unblock the duct. Your baby's sucking will also help, so let him suck even if it's uncomfortable – and expressing is useful too. You could also try a different breastfeeding position, which sometimes helps to unblock a stubborn blocked duct – try the rugby ball position where you put your baby under your arm with just his head peeping out at your breast.

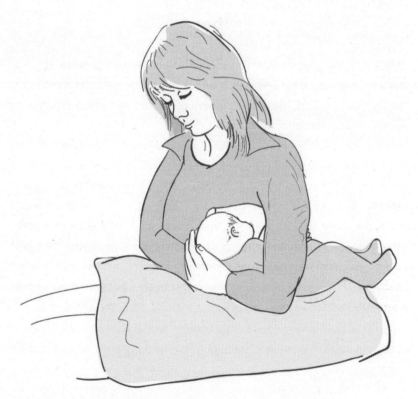

For the rugby ball feeding position you put your baby under your arm with just his head peeping out at your breast.

Lots of dads will go back to work this week having had their two-week paternity break. This won't be easy because you'll be pretty exhausted and will probably find it hard to focus on your work. Then when you get home in the evening, your baby may be crying because it's the end of the day, and your partner will be desperate for a break. Just console yourself that this won't go on forever. Yes it's going to be tough for a few weeks, then you'll notice that things gradually get easier as your baby cries less and your partner becomes more confident as a mother.

PLANNING AHEAD
BCG injection (for tuberculosis)

Until 2005, BCG was given to schoolchildren when they were 15, but this has been stopped because many areas in the UK now have such low TB rates. Instead, the health authorities are targeting high-rate areas, where they are vaccinating babies.

So if your baby is offered a BCG jab it's probably because you live in an area where the TB rate is high – often an inner city area.

Babies will also be offered the BCG jab if their parents or grand-parents have lived in an area with a high TB rate such as South Asia and some parts of Africa. If you think that there's a chance that your baby may be at risk, then speak to your health visitor about having your baby vaccinated. But unless there is someone living in your house-hold who has TB, your baby is almost certainly safe because this disease is very difficult to catch.

week 3

This week you'll probably go to the baby clinic for the first time. You'll find a chaotic-looking room full of buggies, babies and mums, with everyone trying to get their baby undressed and weighed, and their Red Book (see page 47) filled in by a health visitor.

Let the health visitor know that you have arrived so that you get a place in the queue – clinics usually work on a drop-in basis rather than by appointment. And don't forget to bring both the Red Book and also spare nappies as you'll have to completely undress your baby before putting him on the scales.

If for some reason you don't know when or where your local baby clinic is, then give your GP surgery a call. It's important to go to the clinic because as well as having your baby weighed, it gives you the chance to talk through any worries with the health visitor.

Looking after your baby this week will seem a little easier as you are now practised in feeding, bathing and nappy changing. Things generally will seem more under control unless you're unlucky enough to have a colicky baby. Colic, which starts about this time, affects one in 10 babies and results in inconsolable crying in the evenings as your baby experiences painful wind. There are measures you can take to help your baby and reduce his crying (see page 67), but there is no cure as such and parents find colic extremely stressful. So for now it's really a matter of doing what you can to survive the next three months, after which the colic should, in most cases, suddenly disappear.

SLEEP

Total sleep required: 15–18 hours a day
Pattern: irregular

Getting your baby to sleep may have become a bit of an obsession by now and you're bound to have had a go at rocking and sshing him. You'll have noticed that some people have got this down to a real art – they'll take your screaming infant in their arms and somehow calm him and get him off to sleep. But soothing a baby to sleep is something that anyone can learn, it just takes a little patience and practice – and of course your baby mustn't be hungry or you won't stand a chance.

Well-meaning friends and relatives may tell you that you're storing up problems for the future by rocking your baby to sleep, and they may even suggest letting him cry himself to sleep. Ignore them. Mothers have been rocking and singing to their babies since time began, and anyway, it's far too soon to think about 'controlled crying' (where you let your baby cry himself to sleep as part of a sleep training programme).

While rocking your three-week-old infant to sleep is perfectly okay, you can try to avoid letting him become accustomed to anything too elaborate to get him off to sleep – such as climbing up and down the stairs or even a drive around the block. It might be a quickfix solution for the moment, allowing you some much longed for peace, but you don't want to rely on having to take your baby out in the car every night. So try to keep things simple, even if it means that your baby takes slightly longer to settle. This is important because when the time comes for you to back off and allow your baby to soothe himself to sleep, he will find it easier if he's only accustomed to a little gentle rocking.

In the meantime, you can learn the art of calming your baby in your arms as this will be an invaluable tool when your baby is tired, overtired or even ill – any time he needs a little extra help getting to sleep. It's also immensely satisfying to have the skill to be able to soothe your child to sleep. Try the following and see what works for you and your baby, and bear in mind that your partner will develop his own unique method of settling your baby.

Rocking

Gentle movement reminds your baby of being in the womb and definitely speeds up falling asleep. While pregnant you may well have found that your baby was active during the night when you were still, and when you were moving about he seemed to sleep. Well, as far as he's concerned, nothing's changed – he finds it easier to sleep when he's on the move.

So find a carrying position that both you and your baby are comfortable with, then stick with it – his head could rest on your shoulder or in the crook of your arm. Get into a regular rocking rhythm – just pacing up and down a room can be enough movement to soothe your baby – then keep the rhythm going until your baby falls asleep. This could take 20 minutes the first time you try and your baby might well sound more distressed before he begins to settle. But be persistent and try to have confidence that it will eventually work. Keeping an eye on the clock may help because you'll see that what seems like hours of crying is in fact just minutes.

Singing

As well as keeping you relaxed, singing calms your baby as he's familiar with both your voice and your partner's from hearing them while he was in the womb. Babies learn to recognise melodies before they recognise language, and after a few days your baby will start to associate your singing voice with sleep time.

Sshing

To your baby this sounds like the blood pumping to the womb, which can be very reassuring. And it can help release tension when you're desperate for your baby to sleep in the small hours of the morning – you can make quite an angry 'ssh ssh ssh' noise and let out a lot of stress, but your baby will hear only calmness.

Cuddling

Like all babies, your little infant will love being held and cuddled – it's warm, he can smell you, and if you position his head in your left arm (the favoured position for most mums) he will have his ear close to your heart and may even hear it beating.

Patting his bottom

Light, rhythmic pats on your baby's bottom can be soothing as it reminds him of the heartbeat in the womb – that's assuming that he was positioned upside down with his bottom near your heart.

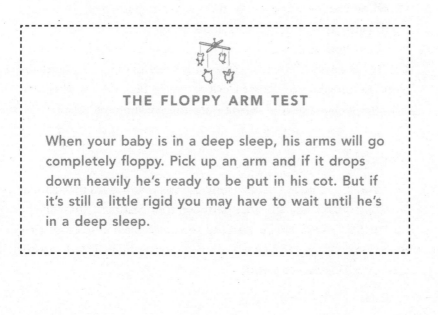

THE FLOPPY ARM TEST

When your baby is in a deep sleep, his arms will go completely floppy. Pick up an arm and if it drops down heavily he's ready to be put in his cot. But if it's still a little rigid you may have to wait until he's in a deep sleep.

SLEEP TRAINING – THE GOLDEN RULE, PUT YOUR BABY DOWN AWAKE

If you want to try some early sleep training, put your baby down when he's calm and sleepy – perhaps because you've been rocking him – but before he's properly asleep. Then watch to see if he manages to settle himself. Teaching your baby to fall asleep is the main factor in sleep training and is the key to eventually having long, peaceful nights.

Start by trying this exercise during the day when you'll have more energy and be able to cope better if your baby wakes up and begins crying after an energy-draining 15 minutes of rocking and singing. Should he start crying then try sshing and resting a comforting hand on his tummy or rocking his crib gently. If this doesn't work then pick him up and start again.

Don't worry if you don't have much luck with this technique because teaching your baby to go to sleep by himself is difficult and something that we shall be returning to time and again over the forthcoming weeks. At this stage, simply getting your baby to go to sleep at all is useful and will help teach him about night and day, and about having naps (see page 200).

CRYING

Number of hours your baby may cry in a day: 1–3
(more than 3 if he's got colic)

You've probably found that your evenings aren't quite what they used to be and that you and your partner end up gobbling your dinner with a crying baby balanced on your lap. Or worse, you have to breastfeed your baby at the table while your partner cuts up your food.

About 9 out of 10 babies will have an unexplained evening crying spell that lasts for between 15 minutes and an hour. No one is sure why babies cry in the evenings, but it could be because they have become wound up from all the excitement during the day and simply need to be soothed. Their anxiety can be exacerbated if you are breastfeeding because your milk supply is at its lowest at the end of the day when you're tired. There isn't a quick fix for evening crying – you have to spend time cuddling, rocking and comfort-feeding your baby (sucking can soothe him). But you will eventually get your evenings back because unexplained crying rarely goes on longer than three months.

Colic

If unexplained crying lasts for longer than three hours and your baby seems to be in extreme pain, drawing up his knees or going rigid, then he has colic. This is when the intestine wall contracts excessively making your baby's tummy taut and painful. Medics define colic as three hours or more of crying, beginning when your baby is three weeks old and occurring for at least three days a week. Colic peaks between weeks 6 and 8 and will disappear by about week 12. But in the meantime, there are steps you can take to soothe your baby that will help both you and your baby to cope.

However stressful you find the crying, rest assured that colic isn't a serious medical condition: your baby will come to no harm and there will be no long-term effects.

If it all gets too much then contact the Cry-sis organisation on 08451 228 669 or go to www.cry-sis.org.uk

A warm bath and a massage

Colic attacks usually occur at the same time each day, so give your baby a bath before a colic attack, not during, to help relax his tummy muscles. You can also massage his tummy before the colic starts with clockwise circles to help the wind through his gut. Generally, massaging during an attack will aggravate him, although all babies are different and some parents say this helps.

Infacol

This colic remedy is available from all chemists and you can give your baby drops throughout the day to help release built-up gas. It's not a miracle cure and some parents say it makes no difference, while others say it helps a little. But it's about the only remedy that is safe to give to a baby from birth. When your baby is a month old you can give him gripe water, which is cheaper than Infacol. Again this isn't a miracle cure – although in the past it was a lot more effective as it contained alcohol. NEVER give your baby alcohol for any reason, including to stop him crying.

Take him for a walk

You can always pack your baby into his buggy so that he will be asleep, or at least be distracted, by the time the colic attack starts. You can also time car journeys around his colic as babies find it almost impossible to stay awake in the car. The main problem with this strategy is that colic tends to peak late in the evening when you won't want to be out pushing the buggy or driving. And you definitely don't want your baby to rely on this, so avoid such a method for more than three consecutive days – enough time for a baby to get into a habit.

Check your feeding technique

If you are breastfeeding then make sure your baby is latching on properly (see page 12) and not gulping air. If bottle-feeding, you could try experimenting with a different style of bottle or teat as some are designed to reduce colic.

Burping

Whether you're breast- or bottle-feeding, it's essential to burp your baby as this helps expel trapped air. Sit him up and rub his back to wind him halfway through a feed for five minutes, and spend time after his feed winding him (see pages 85 and 86). It can take a newborn up to 40 minutes for wind to come up – this will get quicker as your baby gets older and his digestive 'pipes' get bigger to help release more air.

Expelling trapped air

Lie your baby on his back and gently draw his knees up towards his chest – this will sometimes result in releasing trapped wind. Be careful during a colic attack, though, as this could be extremely painful. You can also sit him up and gently bend him forward pushing his nose towards his knees. This can bring up a burp, but again it can be extremely painful for him if he's having a colic attack, so don't do it if it hurts him. Another technique is to lie your baby over your forearm and massage his tummy gently with your other hand.

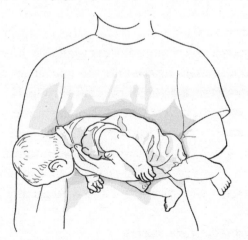

Lie your baby over your forearm and massage his tummy to relieve wind.

Rock him and walk around with him

This is probably what you will end up doing for most of your baby's colic attacks to help him through his painful spasms. Try wearing a baby carrier round the house as this will free up your hands. If your baby doesn't like being rocked, try lying down with him on your tummy while you stroke his back.

Make sure your partner (or anyone else) is around to help with the rocking and soothing as it can be exhausting both physically and emotionally. You could also think about employing someone to come and help – even a babysitter once a week would ease the strain – you could get him or her to take your baby out in the buggy for a couple of hours.

Wear ear plugs or use a personal music player

There's no doubt that listening to your baby screaming when there's little you can do to help him is stressful. Ear plugs or listening to a portable music player will take the edge off the noise, which will help you to stay a little calmer – he will sense that you are less anxious when you hold him.

Cranial osteopathy

This is a gentle and safe treatment that is supposed to release tension in your baby's body resulting from a traumatic birth. Many parents agree that this can be helpful, but few would say it is a miracle cure. Look in your nearest health-food store for contact details of a registered local cranial osteopath or visit www.osteopathy.org.uk.

FEEDING

Total milk required: 600–750 ml/20–25 oz a day
(up to 120 ml/4 oz per feed)
Pattern: 7–10 feeds a day

Don't worry if your baby still doesn't show much sign of settling into a three-hourly feeding pattern – he's very young and the more important issue is still his weight gain. It's important to take your baby along to the clinic in the early months because weight gain is objective and measurements can sometimes reveal underlying problems. Having said that, it's not unknown for some health visitors to place too much importance on weight patterns – if your baby seems happy, then he's more than likely to be healthy.

Try to avoid becoming obsessed with your child's growth – it's quite common for mums to get a bit paranoid and start weighing their babies on the kitchen scales. Most babies put on between 113–170 g/4–6 oz a week for the first six months, but few will grow in a consistent pattern that plots a neat line on the chart – a drift to a different centile over the weeks is very common. The following section explains when to worry about your baby's weight.

Not enough weight gain

Minimal weight gain for a couple of weeks is likely to be just a blip, perhaps if your baby has had a cold and loses his appetite. This is usually followed by a 'catch-up' period during which he'll guzzle extra milk and make up for his previous slow weight gain.

Another reason for slow weight gain at this age is simply that your baby was bigger when he was born than he is genetically programmed to be, so now he is simply finding his true centile on the weight chart. Jumping down one centile really isn't an issue, although most health visitors will start getting a bit anxious if your baby slips down two.

No weight gain

Your baby can go for up to two weeks without gaining weight before it becomes a concern. After two weeks you should definitely seek advice because he's probably not feeding properly and may even be getting dehydrated. Although upsetting, problems with feeding in the early weeks are very common, particularly in breastfed babies. But you will almost certainly be able to sort this out over the next couple of weeks with the help of your health visitor.

Weight loss

If your baby loses weight relatively fast then it is almost certainly because of dehydration due to problems with feeding – the other likely cause is a bout of gastroenteritis making him vomit and have diarrhoea. Always seek help as this can have quite an impact on a young baby. Slow, steady weight loss over several weeks is actually more serious and can indicate heart problems.

Too much weight gain

Your baby may put on a massive 340 g/12 oz a week for a fortnight – again this isn't a problem if it's a one off and your baby seems well. This is generally due to 'catch-up growth' when your baby guzzles a lot of milk after being unwell with, say, a cold. But if your baby is putting on excessive weight and seems unwell then he should be seen by a doctor because he may be retaining too much fluid, which can indicate heart failure.

YOUR BABY'S FINAL SIZE

At this early stage, your baby's position on the weight charts and his growth pattern is no prediction of his final size. A more accurate predictor is the size of you and your partner. But from three months the weight chart can indicate future problems with obesity and give a clearer idea of how big your child will be as an adult.

Breastfeeding

If you want your baby to be able to take a bottle at some stage, then it's a good idea to start this week. He's still young enough to take it without a fuss, but in a few weeks' time you may find that he refuses a bottle. Plenty of breastfeeding mums have struggled unsuccessfully to get their five-month-old babies to take a bottle when they long for a night out, or for their partner to give a night feed.

Giving your baby a bottle now is effortless – you can offer him either expressed milk or formula, and he only needs a couple of ounces, just enough to get him into a sucking rhythm. To keep the habit up, give your baby a bottle every third day.

Bottle-feeding

So far you've been feeding your baby on demand, but you may have asked yourself how you can be sure that you're not feeding him too much. The easiest clue is his weight chart – if your baby falls within the norm and doesn't show any sudden weight increases then you're not overfeeding him.

Another way to check that your baby isn't feeding too much is to watch him while he feeds. When he's had enough he'll turn his head from the bottle and not seem interested so don't be tempted to force him to drink more than he wants or to make him finish his bottle.

If he falls asleep towards the end of his bottle but continues to suck in a light, dreamy way, it means that he's had enough to eat and is just enjoying the comfort. Remove the bottle and see if he'll go to sleep – if he protests too much then let him suck on your finger. Signs that you've given him too much formula include excessive spitting up, and abdominal pain – he will draw his legs up and cry.

NAPPIES

Number of wet nappies over 24 hours: 6–10
Number of dirty nappies over 24 hours: 0–10

Nappy changing will continue to take up a great proportion of your time this week as your baby's bowels remain relentlessly overactive and unpredictable. This makes going out quite difficult as you may well find yourself having to change pooey, and often leaky, nappies in all sorts of places. So if you haven't already got one, buy a travel changing mat – essential for the times you are changing your baby on the floor of a public toilet.

Even if you find a mother and baby changing room, it's not a good idea to put your baby on the shared changing mat. This is because tummy bugs and diarrhoea can be transferred by infected stools on the mat on to your baby's hand – which he then sucks. For the first three months your baby's immune system is immature, and using your own mat reduces his risk of picking up a bug.

WASHING

Nail cutting

Cutting your baby's fingernails can be quite stressful at first as his fingers are so tiny. But his fingernails will grow very fast and need to be trimmed at least once a week so that he doesn't scratch his face. The easiest way is to bite your baby's nails – they are very soft and biting them will ensure that you don't accidentally cut his fingers.

If this doesn't work for you, wait until your baby is asleep and use baby nail scissors (these have blunt ends). Begin by pulling each finger pad back before cutting as this makes the nail seem longer and reduces your chances of cutting his finger. Make sure that you don't leave any sharp corners on his nails which he could scratch himself with. Some mums find baby nail clippers easier to use, although these are extremely sharp so take care.

Scratch mittens are useful when your baby is due for a nail trim but you haven't yet had the chance. If you do cut your baby's finger, don't feel too guilty as this is very common and a baby's skin repairs itself much faster than an adult's. Just dab any blood with a clean tissue and leave it to heal.

Don't worry too much about your baby's toenails – he won't scratch himself with them and they don't grow as fast as fingernails so will only need trimming every few weeks. Sometimes toenails become surrounded by the nail pad making them look ingrown. Use your fingernail to lift your baby's toenail away from his nail pad before trimming, or if this is too difficult simply leave well alone – newborns don't actually suffer from ingrown toenails.

DEVELOPMENT AND PLAYING

Your baby already knows how to wave his arms and will begin to do this more energetically. He is also starting to reach for things with his fists (he's too young to have control over his fingers). When he reaches, he'll do it slowly and probably not hit his target very often.

Although your baby recognises your smell, voice and face, he still only sees your outline (he's a few weeks off being able to pay attention to your features). So if you were to get a drastic haircut, he'd be very confused. Even putting your hair in a ponytail or wearing a hat will make it more difficult for him to recognise you.

Your baby's movements are involuntary but crucial for development. Every time he moves, his brain's messaging system becomes more developed as he learns to link the feel of an object, say your finger in his palm, with what it looks like and where his hand is in space. When enough of these messages have eventually been fired around his brain, he'll understand when he's got something in his hand.

!SAFETY TIP OF THE WEEK!
Warming milk

When warming formula or expressed milk, be extremely careful if using the microwave. Lots of health visitors and midwives will tell you never to use the microwave but to place the bottle in a bowl of hot water instead. This is because microwaving can result in pockets of extremely hot milk that could burn your baby. But if you always remember to shake the bottle well and test the milk's temperature on your wrist, it should be safe.

WHEN TO SEE A DOCTOR

Reflux

It is normal for babies to bring up small amounts of milk – known as possetting – because the valve in between the stomach and the oesophagus (the tube linking the mouth to the stomach) is still undeveloped and weak. If your baby is gaining weight and seems untroubled by the regurgitation, don't worry – even if he seems like a particularly 'sicky' baby and brings up what looks like nearly all his feed (it's easy to overestimate what your baby brings up). He should outgrow reflux by about seven months when the valve develops and strengthens, he spends less time on his back as he learns to sit up, and when he starts eating solids. In the meantime, you can reduce your laundry by using bibs and always having a muslin cloth to hand.

Some babies, however, are extremely troubled by reflux and seem to bring up a lot more milk and to be sensitive to burning acid coming up from the stomach. Severe reflux can make feeding painful, resulting in a lack of weight gain. It can also cause inflammation and bleeding of the oesophagus. So if your baby isn't putting on enough weight, or if his vomit is bloodstained, then see your GP. Be aware that spitting up blood can also occur if you are breastfeeding and have sore, bleeding nipples.

Meticulous winding, lots of small feeds and propping up the head end of your baby's cot can all help. And you can try putting him in a padded bouncy baby chair. Your doctor may also prescribe an antacid such as infant Gaviscon, which reduces acid reflux. If there's no improvement, your GP may arrange for a referral to hospital to perform a pH study, which measures how much acid is being regurgitated. Once the diagnosis has been confirmed in hospital, your baby may be given a drug to speed up the emptying of the stomach or even to reduce acid production. It is usually possible to treat reflux successfully.

In the meantime, be aware that reflux usually begins in the first few weeks, although sometimes it doesn't occur until after three months. Generally, reflux peaks at around four months and improves at seven months, completely disappearing by a year in most children.

WHAT'S HAPPENING TO MUM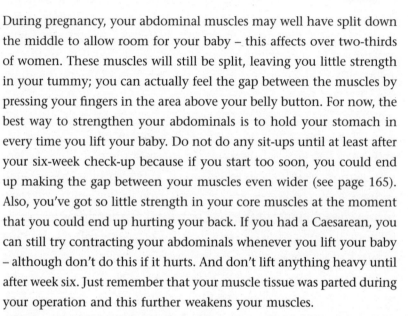

During pregnancy, your abdominal muscles may well have split down the middle to allow room for your baby – this affects over two-thirds of women. These muscles will still be split, leaving you little strength in your tummy; you can actually feel the gap between the muscles by pressing your fingers in the area above your belly button. For now, the best way to strengthen your abdominals is to hold your stomach in every time you lift your baby. Do not do any sit-ups until at least after your six-week check-up because if you start too soon, you could end up making the gap between your muscles even wider (see page 165). Also, you've got so little strength in your core muscles at the moment that you could end up hurting your back. If you had a Caesarean, you can still try contracting your abdominals whenever you lift your baby – although don't do this if it hurts. And don't lift anything heavy until after week six. Just remember that your muscle tissue was parted during your operation and this further weakens your muscles.

Exhaustion can really kick in this week. The 'high' of the birth may have given you energy in the first few weeks, but now you've had over three weeks of very little sleep. There are two things that can help. Firstly, try to get a daytime nap of at least an hour and a half – you may have to arrange for relatives or friends to take your baby during the day so that you can shut the bedroom door and sleep. Do this for two days and you will feel much better. Secondly, try to get four hours of unbroken sleep at night. Just one four-hour session will make a big difference to your mental state. It may mean leaving your partner with the baby in the Moses basket, a bottle and a pile of nappies while you go to bed at 8pm. But do whatever it takes to try and get those four hours.

Post-natal psychosis can occur around now. Also known as puerperal psychosis, this is different from post-natal depression (see page

93), and early signs include being unable to sleep and feeling very restless. You may also have hallucinations, think that no one likes you, and swing from being depressed to being manic. Threatening to harm yourself or your baby is another symptom, but it's unlikely that you will realise that anything is wrong. The condition is specifically pregnancy related and affects about one in 500 new mums, often who have no history of mental illness. You will definitely need psychiatric help and medication, and will be treated in hospital where you will probably stay with your baby. The condition can be treated in weeks, although sometimes it can take a few months to make a full recovery.

For more information see www.mind.org.uk.

PLANNING AHEAD
Naming your baby

Make sure you've agreed on a name for your baby, and don't forget a middle name. You've probably done this already, but plenty of couples are still dithering about names even as they arrive at the registry office to register their child.

week 4

This week, the big event is registering your baby to make him official. You legally have 42 days to register your baby after the birth (21 days in Scotland) – so if you haven't done this yet, time is running out. The baby's father will have to attend if you're not married and he wants his name on the birth certificate – if you're married then you don't have to go together, either one of you is fine.

Registration takes place in your local registry office, which is usually in the town hall – contact your local council for details. You usually don't have to book (you can phone to check) and once you've waited your turn, the whole process only lasts about 10 minutes. There's no need to take any paperwork, just your baby and the following information: his name; sex; the date, time and place of his birth. The registrar will give you a short birth certificate free of charge, which you will need to claim child benefit, and you'll also be given a form for registering your baby at the doctor's. A longer, more detailed birth certificate is available for about £10, and you'll need this full birth certificate showing parental details when you apply for a passport for your child. All children in the UK now need their own passport and can no longer be added to their parents' passports.

The other issue to consider this week is a dummy – will you or won't you use one? A lot will depend on your baby and how much he cries, but if you do go down the dummy route, there are a surprising number of benefits to using one (see page 82).

SLEEP

Total sleep required: *14–17 hours a day*
Pattern: *awake in the evenings*

It's unlikely that your baby will be showing any sign of establishing a sleep pattern yet, apart from being wide awake every evening. Now that he's a few weeks old, your baby will probably stay alert until 11 pm, or even later, and if you try to 'put him to bed' say at 7pm, you will end up running in and out of his room for most of the evening as he needs feeding and soothing.

It's less stressful to go with your baby's sleep pattern for the time being. Move his Moses basket into a quiet, dimly lit corner of your living room so that you can put him down if he does happen to get sleepy. But it's more likely that he'll want to be held and fed for most of the evening and that you'll end up with him on your knee while you try to watch TV. Don't feel guilty, just enjoy cuddling him because in a couple of months he'll be tucked up in his cot in the evenings.

Sleep training tip – bedtime

Observe what time your baby finally gets sleepy at night – a 10-minute doze doesn't count – what you're looking for is a deep, milk-satisfied sleep. If this is a similar time for three consecutive nights you have a 'bedtime'. You can now anticipate his bedtime and begin a bedtime routine about 30 minutes earlier. If it's not too late and you can face it, you could do the full bath routine, perhaps even with a relaxing massage. Otherwise, take him into the bedroom for his night feed, keep the lights low and your voice soft – he should get the message after a few nights that this means bedtime.

If your baby has colic then you'll probably have to wait a few more weeks before you can find his bedtime. But hang on in there – you WILL get your evenings back.

CRYING

Number of hours your baby may cry in a day: 1–6

It's normal for a baby to cry more than ever at the moment, and you can expect these bouts of prolonged, intense, unexplained crying to carry on for another few weeks before you see any improvement. After that you can look forward to your baby falling into a more mature pattern – sleeping more peacefully, feeding at regular times and of course crying less. In the meantime, you've got quite a few more hours of crying to get through, which is why a lot of parents succumb to giving their baby a dummy around now, despite previous high-minded intentions.

If your baby's crying is getting too much to cope with, or if he wants to comfort suck constantly if you're breastfeeding, then it's definitely worth considering a dummy. Breastfed babies shouldn't be given a dummy much earlier than this week because it can confuse their latching-on technique and also upset the fine balance between milk demand and supply. However, bottle-fed babies can have a dummy from around week two, as long as feeding and weight gain are satisfactory.

Lots of mums worry that giving their baby a dummy means they are bad parents, and that they will end up with a buck-toothed three-year-old who insists on being clamped to his dummy all day. The truth is that, while there are problems with using a dummy, there are also advantages. Without a dummy, your baby may start to suck his thumb, which is actually worse for his teeth – partly as you have less control over stopping the habit later on. Having said that, some children's dental development remains totally unaffected by long-term thumb or finger sucking as it all depends on the time that they suck and the force of the sucking.

Here's a round-up of the pros and cons of dummies so that you can make up your own mind.

The pros and cons of giving your baby a dummy

Pros

- A dummy is a quick way to pacify a screaming baby, whose breathing will become calmer and more rhythmic as he sucks.
- Young babies like to suck almost constantly because they find it soothing. If you're breastfeeding, a dummy can give you a break.
- Dummies are better for teeth than finger and thumb sucking which can distort oral anatomy. Also sucking a dummy produces more saliva to fight plaque when your baby's teeth come through.
- You can throw a dummy away when it's time to give up the habit – it's a lot more difficult to stop thumb sucking.
- Some studies have shown that dummies reduce the risk of cot death because sucking stops the infant sleeping too deeply. But this is not conclusive.

Cons

- Dummies can lead to crooked teeth and an open bite – a condition in which the front teeth don't touch when the mouth is closed.
- Sucking a dummy can mask hunger so don't give your baby one if he isn't putting on weight satisfactorily.
- Dummies have been shown to increase a baby's risk of ear infections and diarrhoea – so always sterilise dummies to keep them clean.
- Speech development can be affected as babies don't babble if they have a dummy in their mouths – and babbling is the foundation of speech.
- If you give your baby a dummy in the hope of avoiding thumb sucking, he may spit it out and use his thumb anyway.

Avoiding the dummy pitfalls

- Limit dummies just for the times when your baby is crying and he needs to calm down for a sleep. Then remove the dummy just before your baby falls asleep – he may cry when you do this the first few times but it's worth being persistent, otherwise he'll learn to rely on the dummy to fall asleep.
- Buy several dummies and keep them clean – preferably sterilise them along with your baby's bottles.
- Replace dummies that have split.
- Avoid attached ribbons or strings which could get caught around a baby's throat.
- Ensure that you are feeding your baby enough and that his hunger isn't being masked by sucking a dummy.
- Try to only use a dummy for the first 12 weeks when babies like to comfort suck – after this it becomes harder to break habits and weaning your baby off the dummy will be more difficult (see page 168).

UNEXPLAINED CRYING

If your baby has been reasonably placid until now and his crying seems sudden, it could be that he's ill. Check his temperature (above 38°C/100.4°F indicates a fever) along with other warning signs that things aren't right – such as a loss of appetite – then call your GP if you're worried.

FEEDING

Total milk required: 660–840 ml/22–28 oz a day
(up to 120 ml/4 oz per feed)
Pattern: 7–10 feeds a day

By now your baby will be able to drink faster, which means that feeds are more likely to last 40 minutes than an entire hour. The upside of more efficient feeding is that your baby goes for longer between feeds, perhaps up to four hours on occasion. But more rapid drinking can mean he gulps air so will need lots of burping.

If your baby is one of the lucky ones who seems unaffected by swallowed air, you won't need to bother much with burping. Some babies, on the other hand, are very sensitive to wind, in which case you will need to make burping him an essential part of his feeding routine and be very patient while you wait for the air to come up. Small quantities of air swallowed during feeding form tiny bubbles in the stomach that eventually make a large bubble that can be burped up. That's why babies are often windier at the end of the day.

When to burp your baby

You can do this halfway through the feed and then again at the end. Or you can wait until your baby takes a natural pause while feeding and burp him then. Allow five minutes for any air to come up during a feed, or longer if your baby shows signs of discomfort. It can take up to 40 minutes for air to come up once his feed is finished.

Different ways to burp your baby

1. Sit your baby on your knee
   with his chin resting on
   yourfinger and thumb,
   then gently rub his back
   with your other hand. You
   can try tilting him forward
   slightly as this can help to
   expel air – but it can also
   be uncomfortable for your
   baby if he's particularly
   windy so stop as soon as
   he protests.

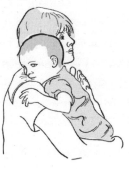

2. Hold your baby upright
   against your chest with his
   head resting on your
   shoulder. Your baby's
   stomach is pressed gently
   against your chest and this
   can encourage air to come
   up – you can also rub his
   back.

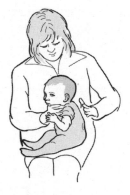

3. Lay your baby on your lap,
   tummy downwards, and
   rub his back. Alternating
   this lying down position
   with the more upright
   burping postures (above)
   seems to encourage wind
   to come up.

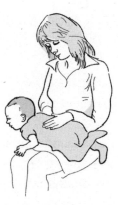

Breastfeeding

By now, breastfeeding is well established and you are probably appreciating this hassle-free choice – you don't have to fiddle around in the middle of the night warming bottles, and if you had painful let down as your milk was released in the early days, this will have subsided. But complications do still occur – nipples can once again get sore as you become less conscientious about perfecting your latch-on technique. Or you may get a bout of mastitis – an infected duct – or perhaps find that your baby decides to only drink from one breast. But as always, there are solutions and it is worth battling through.

Mastitis

Mastitis can occur at any time, although it's quite common around now possibly because your milk production has increased. Mastitis begins as a blocked milk duct so treat this as soon as you become aware of the problem (see page 60). Hot baths, hot flannels, massage and plenty of sucking by your baby should unblock the duct.

If the duct becomes infected, you will need antibiotics, though you can continue to feed throughout treatment. So if a blocked duct shows no improvement after 24 hours, go and see your doctor.

Favourite breast

Another problem that often begins about now is that your baby starts to favour one breast. This usually happens because, like most mums, you find it easier to feed on one side so you'll naturally offer your baby your 'easier' breast, especially if you're out and about and feeling self-conscious about feeding in public. Then of course milk production increases on this side, which encourages your baby to favour that breast, and a pattern is soon established.

Try to break this cycle now before milk production in your non-favoured breast diminishes – lots of women end up lopsided throughout breastfeeding. So offer your baby your non-favoured breast first at every feed, and also pump from this one to increase milk production. It should only take a couple of days to even things out.

Bottle-feeding

You'll be fast and efficient at making up feeds by now, but don't be too hasty when measuring out the scoops of powder and water. It's essential that you use the exact measurements because if the formula is too concentrated it can put a strain on your baby's immature kidneys and gut. Always follow the directions to the letter and don't ever be tempted to 'keep your baby going a little longer' by adding extra milk powder to his feed.

Should your baby get diarrhoea then your doctor may tell you to make up the formula to be more dilute than usual to help prevent dehydration – but you shouldn't do this unless you've had medical advice to do so, and not for more than a few days because your baby won't be getting adequate calories.

NAPPIES

Number of wet nappies over 24 hours: 4–8
Number of dirty nappies over 24 hours: 0–8

At last you should see an improvement in the numbers of nappies you are changing. This week you won't be changing quite so many nappies because your baby will be weeing less as his kidneys are now more developed. And if he has been doing one poo per feed up until now, this should stop by the end of the week as his bowel movements settle down and become less frequent. So you should see an end to changing nappies throughout the night – there's no need to worry if your baby's nappy is a bit wet at night as urine alone won't cause nappy rash.

WASHING

Now that your baby doesn't seem quite so fragile, you could try bathing with him (if you haven't already done so). This is a wonderful bonding experience which you can enjoy with your baby on your chest as you gently slosh water over him.

Have the water a little cooler than you would normally for a bath – the temperature should obviously suit your baby rather than you. And for the first couple of times you'll probably like your partner to be around to pass your baby to you, although it's possible to step into the bath holding him if you have a bath mat to stop you slipping. After the bath you'll need to wear a towelling robe as you won't have time to dry yourself until you've dried and dressed your baby. The best arrangement is for your partner to take your baby out of the bath to be dried, while you top it up with hot water and wallow.

Lots of dads also love bathing with their baby, although they'll probably make a lot of fuss if your baby happens to wee in the water (urine is sterile so this isn't a problem). Thankfully babies rarely, if ever, poo in the bath.

DEVELOPMENT AND PLAYING

This week your baby will start crying his first actual tears, which can be particularly heart-rending. This happens because the glands over the eyeballs start to produce enough fluid for his tears to flow in sufficient quantity; until now he has cried with dry eyes.

Your baby will be kicking more vigorously this week as he learns to use his large muscles – he's building the muscles that will eventually enable him to walk. Already your baby has a stepping reflex and you can make him 'walk' by trying the following: hold him upright under his arms near a table, then manoeuvre him so that the top of the table strokes the top of one of his feet. This triggers his step reflex. Next, quickly hold him so that he is 'standing' on the table and watch his feet take a few steps.

Although your baby still needs to rest his head on your shoulder a lot of the time, he no longer seems quite as floppy and will be able to hold his head up for a few moments. He's gradually building his neck muscles and learning to control them. Babies develop their muscles from their neck downwards, so this muscle control will progress down his body over the next few weeks as he learns to move his arms, strengthen his trunk to sit and finally develop his legs for walking.

Put your baby on his front to 'play' – you can put some toys near his head for him to look at. He may lift his head briefly, and this helps develop his back and shoulder muscles. He'll probably only be happy on his front for a few minutes at a time but persevere because after week six he'll probably refuse to go on his tummy at all. This position is important for physical development as it strengthens his back muscles, particularly as he starts to lift his head. Lying on his back doesn't have the same strengthening benefits, which is why babies nowadays have delayed motor skill development, so they roll over and crawl later than in the past. This isn't a problem and your baby will catch up in the end, but put him on his front as often as possible to counterbalance the hours he spends asleep on his back.

Another advantage of putting your baby on his front is that it reduces his chance of ending up with flattened head syndrome (see page 270). Although harmless, this is much more common now that babies routinely sleep on their backs. Babies can go on their fronts from the day they are born, but parents are reluctant because of the associations with cot death. As long as you are around to ensure he doesn't nod off, there are no safety worries.

You can try having a 'conversation' with your baby as he is now able to make clear vowel sounds such as 'eeh' and 'aah'. If you copy him and make similar sounds you'll find that he responds. One of the functions of all the recent crying was to give him practice at making vowel sounds.

!SAFETY TIP OF THE WEEK!
Scalds

Bath scalds:
When running your baby's bath, always put the cold water in before the hot to avoid accidentally scalding your baby. Babies have thinner skin than adults, making them more susceptible to burns. Because they aren't mobile they won't be able to jump away from the heat and this can make a bathwater scald potentially serious.

Put him straight into cold water for at least 10 minutes and apply ice to the affected skin (a bag of frozen peas wrapped in a muslin cloth works well) – this should make any redness disappear in a few hours. Your baby should be seen within a few hours by your health visitor or GP for all scalds and burns. If this isn't possible then take your baby along to your hospital's Emergency Department if there is still any redness after a couple of hours, or if he seems grizzly with pain.

Hot drink scalds:
Don't drink tea or coffee while holding your baby – drinks can still scald 15 minutes after the kettle has boiled, and your baby is becoming more wriggly by the day.

If you spill a hot drink on your baby remove any wet clothes to expose the burnt area, then treat the scald as above. But if the burn is larger than your baby's hand it means that about 1 per cent of his skin surface area has been damaged, which is potentially dangerous. Take him to hospital as he may well need intravenous fluids, pain relief and possible skin grafts.

WHEN TO SEE A DOCTOR

Pyloric stenosis

This is a rare but serious condition when the outlet to the stomach becomes blocked because the ring of muscle between the stomach and the duodenum thickens. This means that very little milk can leave the stomach, which in turn becomes so full that eventually your baby vomits. Babies with the condition can vomit up nearly an entire meal after just about every feed, and sometimes the vomit will be projected up to a metre across the room. After vomiting, your baby will be very hungry. You'll also notice that bowel movements are infrequent, your baby won't gain weight and that he may start to look emaciated.

Pyloric stenosis is five times more common in boys and usually occurs from now until eight weeks old. Dehydration is the big danger so see your doctor quickly and they will check for the condition by feeling your baby's stomach for swelling during a feed. Your doctor's diagnosis will be confirmed in hospital by an ultrasound scan, then your baby will be given an operation to widen his stomach outlet. He should make a full recovery.

WHAT'S HAPPENING TO MUM

By now, your weight will have stopped dropping off quite so rapidly and begin to settle down. From now onwards, weight loss will require a regular diet and exercise regime, but if you are breastfeeding then don't lose more than a pound a week or your milk production will be affected. Avoid heavy exercise (running, playing squash, lifting big weights at the gym) because your ligaments are still loose and you could end up injured. Pregnancy hormones loosened the ligaments around your pelvis to help get your baby out, but the hormones aren't selective and so all your ligaments were loosened. After about three months your ligaments will be tight enough to avoid most injuries, but it takes up to five months for them to be completely back to normal. The best exercise at the moment is pushing the buggy – you don't need a babysitter and walking burns off about 350 calories an hour.

It's also important to watch your posture, particularly when lifting and cradling your baby, and also while breastfeeding. It's easy to be hunched when you're feeling very tired but this can lead to backache. During pregnancy your spine's curvature became more pronounced to support the weight of your baby. Now, although the curve is becoming less pronounced as the vertebrae are realigned, it can take up to three months to fully return to normal.

If your baby blues never really went away then you could develop post-natal depression (PND) around now, although PND more commonly occurs between four and six months after the birth (see page 212). Your health visitor will probably give you a PND question-naire at nine weeks to pick up any problems (see page 157 for details on this assessment).

PND affects one in 10 women, and having a history of depression increases your chances of suffering. You may experience tearfulness, not enjoying your baby, irritability, insomnia, lack of appetite, anxiety about your baby and concerns about being a bad mother. Mild PND can get better by itself within three to six months, although some-times it can go on for a year. Surprisingly, only one in four mums seek help, but if you feel low most of the time for more than a week speak to your GP or health visitor. You will probably be offered six counselling sessions at your home – 80 per cent of women recover quickly with counselling, the others may be offered antidepressants. For more details see www.mind.org.uk

Lots of dads don't bond with their babies at first. If you're a dad and this sounds like you, it can be particularly hard as you watch your partner gazing at your baby as though he's the most amazing creature in the world. But dads won't feel out of it for much longer because in a couple of weeks your baby will start smiling, then he'll giggle and you'll finally feel that he's actually giving something back. This is when dads and babies really start to bond.

PLANNING AHEAD
Your six-week check

Book your six-week check with your GP – you will need a double appointment as your doctor will want to see both you and your baby. Write down any questions as they come to you between now and your appointment.

If you had a complicated delivery, you will need to be seen by a hospital doctor and should already have been given an appointment – speak to your health visitor if you're unsure. Your baby may still be seen by your GP.

week 5

Your baby is nearly six weeks old and is due for his routine six-week check-up either this week or next to ensure that he's fit and healthy. Take your baby's Red Book so that the doctor can record details, and also bring spare nappies as your baby will have to undress to be weighed. Your doctor will give your baby a thorough all-over check including examining his eyes, ears and mouth, and checking his hips, spine, heart, tummy, genitals, hands and feet.

It's very unlikely that this check-up will reveal anything sinister and the majority of babies get the all-clear. The most likely problem to be discovered during this appointment is a heart murmur, which affects up to one in 100 babies. Any serious heart problems would almost certainly have been revealed by now, so at this stage your baby probably won't have anything worse than a small hole in the heart which may close by itself or might need a small operation.

The other problem that may show up at this check-up is congenital dislocation of the hips, which affects around one in 1,000 babies – again this is straightforward to correct, usually with surgery and/ or plastering.

The doctor will ask you questions about your baby's feeding, whether he is smiling yet and if he turns towards light and is startled by loud noises. This information helps the doctor make a developmental assessment. It's also a good opportunity for you to ask questions if you have any concerns. If your baby is given a clean bill of health, he won't have another routine health check until he is eight months and will now only see the doctor if he has something specifically wrong with him.

You too will have your six-week check and hopefully will also be signed off, which means that you and your baby are now officially out of the midwifery and obstetrics health system. Of course, your doctor will still be accommodating should you have any worries, so don't ever worry about 'bothering' the GP if you're concerned about your baby. When booking the appointment, tell the receptionist your baby's age and you'll probably be seen within 24 hours. Doctors take baby illnesses seriously because babies can deteriorate rapidly and are vulnerable.

SLEEP

Total sleep required: 14–17 hours a day
Pattern: sleeps more at night than during the day

Your baby's sleep pattern will still seem pretty random, although you'll notice that he's beginning to sleep for longer stretches at night as he begins to differentiate between night and day. This is the first stage of learning to eventually sleep through the night, but it's a long slow process and right now your sleep continues to be broken. What's particularly hard is that you can't yet have an early night when you're feeling exhausted because your baby is almost certainly still crying and needing lots of feeds in the evenings.

Sleeping with your baby

Around now lots of mums become so desperate for sleep that they guiltily tuck their baby into their own bed at night as a last resort to get a few hours of rest. Current NHS guidelines state that the safest place for your baby to sleep is in a cot in your room. But research shows that if you're not a drinker or smoker and you take precautions (see page 100), the risk of bed sharing is radically reduced. Dad must abstain too, or sleep on the couch.

If you've ever dropped off to sleep while breastfeeding your baby only to wake with a start hours later, you're certainly not alone. It's estimated that up to 40 per cent of mothers in the Western world sleep with their babies (figures are higher in other cultures), and it's even more prevalent among breastfeeding mums who don't have to get out of bed to feed. Just make absolutely sure that you follow the safe bed sharing guidelines.

It's believed that if you're breastfeeding and you sleep with your baby then you become tuned in with your baby's sleep cycles after a few nights as you both fall in and out of sleep together and both become semi-awake as your baby feeds. This sounds like a blissfully straightforward solution to sleep deprivation for new mothers, and it is for many cultures around the world.

But if you've tried sleeping with your baby, or are considering it, you will no doubt be plagued by worry that you might accidentally smother him to death. Statistically the chances of this happening are incredibly rare – in the UK around 300 babies die of cot death (Sudden Infant Death Syndrome) per year. Of these, less than 1 per cent die of suffocation in their parents' bed. And these deaths can be avoided according to a population study published in the *British Medical Journal* in 1999. This research found that there was no association of death through suffocation if parents didn't smoke, avoided alcohol, didn't fall asleep on the sofa with the baby (squashier than a bed so more likely to suffocate a baby), weren't extremely tired and the baby didn't get trapped under the quilt. Although most new parents would describe themselves as 'extremely tired' you only need to worry if you feel too tired to leave the house – if this happens, don't sleep with your baby.

So provided that you take precautions, sleeping with your baby appears to be safe. And, what's more, there's even evidence it is beneficial for your child. Of all the mammals, humans are born the most neurologically immature and so need close human contact for basic survival. Some studies have claimed that children who slept with their parents do better at school, are less stressed and more confident. Whether or not you co-sleep is a very personal choice and there are many variations on sharing a bed with your baby. Whatever you decide, it has to be a joint decision made with your partner that you both feel happy about.

Some parents opt to share their bed from day one and continue to do so until their baby is about three and (hopefully) chooses to sleep by himself. Others never have their baby in their bed, even for night feeds because mum sits in a chair to feed her infant. But a lot of parents fall somewhere in between. They put their baby to bed in his own cot, then when he wakes in the night mum will take him into bed for a feed and keep him there for a few hours or until the morning. She might do this every night or just a couple of times a month, or perhaps when he has a cold and isn't sleeping well. Another option is to buy a cot which has one open side, designed to attach to the side of an adult bed. Again this teaches your baby to sleep separately from you, while also allowing him to snuggle up for night feeds without having to wake up fully.

If you are thinking about sleeping with your baby then one fundamental question you should ask yourself is how you would cope if your baby were to die from cot death while in your bed. Would you be plagued by guilt and regret despite the fact that your baby's death was highly unlikely to have been caused by bed sharing? And bear in mind that even a verdict of accidental death can end up in the newspapers as a shock news piece accompanied by quotes from experts advising parents not to sleep with their babies. Some NHS midwives and health visitors will happily advise on safe co-sleeping, but Western society at large is still wary of bed sharing with babies. And this in itself makes the decision about whether to take your baby into your bed ever more complicated.

HOW TO AVOID ENDING UP WITH A FIVE-YEAR-OLD IN YOUR BED

If you want to bed share but don't want your baby to still be in your bed when he's older, then follow these two basic rules to avoid bad habits.

Firstly, don't let him use you as a 'human dummy' when you breastfeed him. Your baby will think this is wonderful and won't want to go back to sleeping by himself. So when he's finished his feed, take him off your breast, or, better still, put him back in his cot even if he makes a fuss.

Secondly, always let your baby fall asleep by himself in his cot – plenty of parents end up in a situation where the only way to get their baby to sleep is to lie with him on the bed for 20 minutes patiently cuddling him while he drifts off.

Sleeping safely with your baby

- Never share your bed with your baby if you or your partner smoke.
- Don't sleep with your baby if you or your partner have been drinking alcohol or taking drugs.
- Don't sleep with your baby if you are suffering from extreme exhaustion.
- Don't share your bed with your baby if you or your partner are obese.
- Don't sleep with your baby in a waterbed or on a deep-pile mattress cover – make sure your mattress is firm.
- Don't fall asleep with your baby on a sofa – babies can get trapped in the awkward corners and squashy sofas can suffocate.
- Use a minimum number of pillows and keep them well away from your baby.
- Don't let your baby become covered by the duvet – using just a cotton sheet is the safest option, otherwise keep the duvet tucked well away from your baby's head.
- Don't place your baby between yourself and the wall as he may slip down the bed and get trapped.
- Ensure that there isn't a gap between the mattress and the head-board in which your baby could get trapped and suffocate.
- Don't take your baby into bed if he is wearing a baby sleeping bag or he'll get too hot.
- Remove any buttons from your nightdress that your baby may 'suck' on during the night – at the very least check that they aren't loose.
- Don't let your baby sleep on his tummy, although sleeping on your chest is okay as babies have been shown to mimic their mothers' breathing thus reducing their cot death risk.
- Don't leave your baby alone in the adult bed – he may fall out.
- Don't put pillows around the bed to cushion him should he fall out of bed – he may suffocate in them.
- Tell your partner that your baby is in the bed – it's important

that he's always aware of your baby's presence, particularly if you take your baby into bed in the middle of the night.

CRYING

Number of hours your baby may cry in a day: 1–6

The amount your baby cries will continue to increase as he revs up for his big crescendo next week. As you listen to all this wailing, you may notice that his cries have different meanings, and as you gradually learn to distinguish them over the next few weeks you'll be rewarded by a marked decrease in how much he cries.

Different cries

Hunger – rhythmic and relentless, this crying will go on and on with barely a pause; nothing will stop this cry apart from milk, so if your baby is hungry then feed him.

Pain – high pitched, almost as though your baby is screaming out in pain. You may hear this when your baby has wind, he has his vaccinations, or if you accidentally bend his arm backwards while dressing him. Try to learn this cry as soon as possible so that you can recognise it when your baby cries out about more serious causes of pain.

Tiredness – lots of variation: strong and determined cries fade to a grizzle, with intermittent silent pauses. Crying from overtiredness will become increasingly prevalent in the coming weeks.

Emotional – this covers anything from your baby feeling bored with sitting in the same place, frightened because a loud noise has made him jump, angry because he wants to be picked up and cuddled, or feeling frustrated because his milk runs out halfway through a feed. Emotional crying is sometimes accompanied by your baby sticking his lip out, making him look petulant. Emotional crying is more difficult to recognise as there are variations between babies, but it can sometimes sound as though your baby is doing a fake cry and putting it on for effect – he's not and he feels genuinely emotional.

FEEDING

Total milk required: *660–900 ml/22–30 oz a day (up to 135 ml/4½ oz per feed)*
Pattern: *7–10 feeds a day*

When your baby was born, it was essential that he was fed on demand, around the clock, and you probably gave him lots of tiny feeds. But now his stomach is bigger and he can go for longer without milk. Most babies will wait for three hours during the day between feeds (remember that this is three hours from the start of one feed to the start of the next) and four hours at night. If your baby still loves his constant, tiny feeds, then try the following to help him break this habit – your life will seem a lot easier, particularly at night.

Breastfeeding

If you are still feeding more than every two hours, it could be that your baby isn't having a full feed. Remember that breast milk changes during a feed – at first your baby will receive fore milk, which is sweet, watery and thirst quenching, high in milk sugar but low in fat. This gives him instant hydration and energy. As the feed goes on, richer hind milk is released, which is higher in fat and calories.

So it's important to be patient and let your baby completely finish drinking from one breast before swapping him over, if indeed you do. Otherwise don't put him on the other breast until the next feed. Allow him to feed from one breast for at least 20 minutes and watch as his sucking slows down and he becomes dopey and relaxed. This means that he has reached the hind milk, which makes him more likely to go for longer until his next feed.

Bottle-feeding

If your baby doesn't want much of his bottle and you find that you are still throwing away a lot of milk, it could be that he's got into the habit of grazing – having lots of small feeds throughout the day and night. Apart from wasting a lot of milk, this is particularly hard going at night.

By now your baby should be drinking as much as 135 ml/4½ oz during some feeds. If you think that your baby is grazing and you want to make some changes, begin by working on his daytime feeding habits. You'll have more energy during the day and changes he makes will have a knock-on positive effect at night.

Start by making your baby wait an extra five minutes for a feed and see how he reacts. If he doesn't mind too much then extend this to 10 and so on until he is going three hours between feeds, then you can gradually work on him going for four hours at night. Don't be too regimented at this stage and be aware of what your baby is telling you. If he's saying that he's really not ready to wait this long between feeds then let him have his way – you can always try this again in a couple of weeks.

NAPPIES

Number of wet nappies over 24 hours: 4–8
Number of dirty nappies over 24 hours: 0–8

It's quite common for both breastfed and bottle-fed babies to push, strain and go red in the face when going to the toilet even though their poos are very soft. This is thought to be because the anus muscles aren't very good at relaxing yet, and also because babies tend to go to the toilet lying down so don't get the benefit of gravity. Excessive straining tends to settle down by about week 10. Be aware that babies can become constipated, which explains straining – and this needs treating (see page 116).

WASHING

Cradle cap

This is when your baby's scalp becomes crusty with patches of yellow-brown greasy flakes. Although it looks unpleasant, it won't bother your baby because it isn't itchy or sore. It's unlikely to persist beyond six months.

Treating cradle cap

You can give your baby a gentle head massage with olive oil before his bath, then brush his 'hair' however little he has, to help dislodge the scales (use a soft baby brush). Wash the oil off with baby shampoo as this may also help to dislodge the scales.

Tea tree oil is known to be effective in treating cradle cap, so add a few drops to four tablespoons of olive oil and rub this on to your baby's scalp at bedtime, then shampoo off in the morning. You could also mix a few drops of tea tree oil with your baby's shampoo.

If your baby's cradle cap is particularly stubborn, use a medicated cradle cap shampoo (available from the chemist). Or your doctor can prescribe a mild topical steroid if the problem is very persistent. NEVER pick at the scales – however tempting.

DEVELOPMENT AND PLAYING

If you move an object from side to side above your baby's head, he will now be able to follow it with his eyes. This is because his brain has developed to anticipate an object's movement allowing him to track it.

Limit the time that your baby sits in a car seat because these are very rigid and restrict a baby's movement, resulting in less muscle development. The worst thing you can do is transport your baby in and out of the car in one of these seats and keep him in it for hours on end. When you're at home it's better to put your baby in a specifically designed bouncy baby seat that allows him to wriggle around and in doing so use his muscles. The best option of all is to put your baby on his front on the floor when he's awake, and the next best choice is to place him on his back – both these positions develop his muscles.

> **! SAFETY TIP OF THE WEEK !**
> **Never clean bottle teats with salt**
>
> Lots of parents make the mistake of washing bottle teats with salty water to get them clean. But you should never ever do this because it's difficult to rinse all the salt off properly, and your baby ends up ingesting it. His kidneys are still far too immature to excrete it and salt levels in the blood can rise to dangerously high levels – which are potentially lethal.

WHEN TO SEE A DOCTOR

Thrush

If your baby becomes inexplicably difficult to feed and seems irritable, then it's possible he has oral thrush. This is quite common in new babies and some babies even catch it during birth from their mothers, particularly if the mother suffered from vaginal thrush during pregnancy.

Thrush is a fungal infection caused by *Candida albicans* and thrives in warm damp conditions, so can affect the vagina, mouth, nipples during breastfeeding and the nappy area. Oral thrush can make your baby's mouth sore, which is why feeding can be difficult. Look for white spots on his tongue and inside his cheeks – if you wipe these with a tissue they probably won't dislodge, and if they do they will expose a red, sore patch. Thrush can also cause persistent nappy rash which is bright red and doesn't respond to usual nappy rash treatment – you may also notice white patches on the skin.

It's important to see your doctor if you suspect your baby has thrush as this is a fungal infection that requires treatment. Your doctor will prescribe anti-fungal drops to put in your baby's mouth after feeds, plus an anti-fungal cream to apply to his nappy area – leaving your baby without a nappy will help to speed up healing. The condition usually responds after a couple of days of treatment and it's essential that you continue medication after symptoms have disappeared to prevent a recurrence.

If you are breastfeeding then you should also treat your nipple area with an anti-fungal cream after every feed – pain after feeds is likely if you have thrush on your nipples.

WHAT'S HAPPENING TO MUM

The six-week check marks your official discharge from the maternity services as long as there are no complications. You'll probably be seen by your GP unless you had a complicated delivery, in which case you will be seen by a hospital doctor. The doctor will feel your tummy to make sure that your uterus has returned to its pre-pregnant size. She will also do a urine test to check for infections and diabetes, and will check for high blood pressure, which can sometimes occur as a result of pregnancy. Finally your doctor will check your episiotomy scar, if you had one.

This is a good opportunity to mention to your doctor if your baby blues haven't lifted yet as this could indicate post-natal depression (see page 93). You can also mention if your stitches are still sore as this shouldn't be the case, and tell the doctor if sex is difficult or if you haven't yet been able to face it.

If you've not yet had sex then you certainly aren't unusual because a lot of women choose to wait several months after giving birth, partly because they're afraid it will hurt. Sex shouldn't be painful unless you have particularly bad scarring, so speak to your doctor if sex is uncomfortable after the first few times.

The prospect of getting pregnant again can also put women off sex, so speak to your doctor about contraception (see page 108). Another common worry is that sex won't be as good because your vagina will be 'bigger' – again this won't be an issue as the vagina is designed to be extremely elastic and by six weeks will have returned to pre-pregnancy size. You can continue with your pelvic floor exercises (see page 45) to tighten the muscles.

Some women worry that they won't enjoy sex as much – again this is a myth as it probably won't be any different and lots of women say it's actually better because they feel closer to their partner having had a child. A few women even say that they reach orgasm more easily, which is thought to be because blood supply to the genitals increases after childbirth.

But the main reason for not wanting sex yet is usually exhaustion combined with your hormones still being all over the place, reducing libido. Be patient – your sex life will return, and in the meantime don't be embarrassed to mention any concerns to your doctor or health visitor who will have dealt with this problem time and time again.

It's also important to talk to your partner about how you feel – explain to him that lots of women go off sex for a while but that your sex drive should return before too long. The more patient and understanding he is, the more quickly you're likely to want sex again.

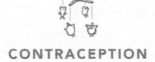

CONTRACEPTION

If you're not breastfeeding, you may get your period any time from now. It's essential that you speak to your GP about contraception because you will be fertile two weeks before menstruation.

If you're breastfeeding, don't rely on it for contraception – it doesn't work. If you used to take the pill you will now have to consider other forms of contraception because the combined pill contains oestrogen (as well as progesterone) and this interferes with milk production. Lots of breastfeeding women opt for the mini pill which only contains progesterone so doesn't upset lactation. The downside is that it isn't as reliable. Discuss the pros and cons with your doctor.

Other options include a diaphragm, although you'll need to be re-fitted now that you've given birth. And lots of couples choose to use condoms until the woman has finished breastfeeding and goes back on the pill.

PLANNING AHEAD
Book your post-natal exercise classes

Some of the larger hospitals run exercise classes for mums in their early post-natal period. Mums can attend six weeks after a vaginal delivery and eight to ten weeks after a Caesarean delivery – so it might be worth calling the hospital where you had your baby to see what's available. If your hospital doesn't provide such classes, you could enquire about post-natal yoga and Pilates in your area – although you'll have to pay for these classes. You can also go to www.postnatalexercise.co.uk to find a teacher in your area who does general exercise classes for new mums.

Alternatively, just walking with the pram is great exercise. Walking burns around 350 calories an hour so if you aim to eventually do at least an hour a day, and to speed up until you feel slightly out of breath, you won't need to join a gym to get back in shape.

week 6

This week you will probably see your baby's first big milestone – his first real smile. You may have had glimpses of smiles over the last few weeks as you watched your newborn grinning away in his sleep or as he forced out some wind. Although exciting, these early smiles will soon pale into insignificance once you've witnessed a social smile, when your baby looks you in the eye and grins away because he's happy.

This is a rewarding week for parents as your baby undergoes tremendous developmental advances. You'll see him change from a strange little creature trapped in his own bubble – only really aware of his hunger and wind – to a real little person who is suddenly curious about people and his surroundings. But this is also a tough week because your baby's crying will be peaking, he'll be going through a growth spurt and from now onwards he'll start to fight sleep and become overtired – adding another challenge to the sleeping conundrum.

SLEEP

Total sleep required: 14–17 hours a day
Pattern: sleeps more at night than during the day – aim for daytime naps that total at least three hours

As your baby becomes more sociable, he'll start to resist falling asleep because he'd rather stay awake and play. So instead of dropping off to sleep when he's tired, full of milk and winded, your baby will actually fight sleep because he's excited about his newly discovered world. The result is that he can end up extremely overtired.

At night your baby's needs will be simple to meet because you can be sure that he's tired, even if he seems desperate to stay awake. But during the day it's easy to let your baby stay awake for too long. And once he becomes overtired, it actually gets harder for him to fall asleep because he feels more and more wound up and over-emotional. It might seem logical to keep your baby awake all day so that he's exhausted by bedtime and sleeps more at night, but it doesn't work like that. Your baby should have at least three hours' sleep during the day or he will feel so tired and over-emotional that night sleep will be disrupted. Remember how you feel after a stressful day – your head buzzes and although you're exhausted there's no way you feel like sleeping. So it's important to watch for cues that he's tired and put him down to sleep before he becomes exhausted.

SIGNS THAT YOUR BABY IS TIRED

- yawning
- rubbing his eyes
- pulling his ears
- grizzling
- avoiding eye contact

When to put your baby down for a daytime nap

Babies of this age will become tired after they've been awake for two hours – so if you make sure that you put your baby down for a sleep when he's been up for a couple of hours he won't become fractious, tearful or too tired to settle calmly to sleep. You'll find it difficult to get your baby into a napping routine (see page 200) while he's still so young, especially as you're unlikely to have got a bedtime established yet. But if you aim for him to have at least three hours of daytime sleep, this is a good start. Eventually he'll have a more defined napping pattern of three naps a day – one early morning, a longer sleep at lunchtime then finally a short sleep in the late afternoon.

CRYING

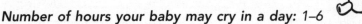

Number of hours your baby may cry in a day: 1–6

At six weeks of age your baby's crying will peak before slowly starting to improve from next week onwards. The reason babies cry so much this week is thought to be tied in with them making monumental developmental advances, such as smiling and interacting, which require a lot of energy and concentration. Your baby quickly becomes exhausted and tearful.

This huge leap coincides with your baby's six-week growth spurt, so if he is breastfed, he may go a bit short of milk this week – giving him another good reason to cry. And if he's bottle-fed he'll also need extra milk to fuel his growth spurt, which he'll demand by crying. To complicate things further, your baby will now start to cry for a new reason – overtiredness. As a newborn he would have simply gone to sleep as soon as he felt tired, but now that your baby is older he will fight sleep, which will leave him feeling fractious and tearful as he becomes more and more tired. An overtired baby can often get quite muddled about what's actually upsetting him and may cry to be fed because he's feeling upset and wants comfort, not because he's hungry. So guessing why your baby is crying becomes ever more confusing. The key to preventing overtired crying is to put your baby down for a nap before he reaches exhaustion point. Because you probably won't have your baby on any sort of routine at the moment, the failsafe way is to offer him food when he starts grizzling and if he's not interested then put him down for a nap.

FEEDING

Total milk required: 660–900 ml/22–30 oz a day
(up to 150 ml/5 oz per feed)
Pattern: 6–10 feeds a day, your baby's growth spurt may mean
even more frequent feeding than usual

Your baby is due for another growth spurt this week and it will probably be even bigger than the last one, so expect him to be ravenous. He'll be stoking up on extra energy to fuel his developmental milestones such as smiling and interacting. As you found during his last growth spurt, he may become bad tempered, particularly if you are breastfeeding and he's not getting enough milk. It's quite common to think that you've 'lost' your milk but this isn't the case. It's just the coincidence of your baby making extra demands and your breasts softening at around this time as your milk production settles. Again, breastfeed around the clock to allow your supply to increase to match your baby's demand. And whether your baby is being breast- or bottle-fed, hunger will be a big reason for his tears this week. Growth spurts usually last a couple of days, after which your baby will seem more settled. And he may even drop a feed because he is now able to take more milk at each meal.

Breastfeeding – alcohol

You've probably wondered how much alcohol you can drink while breastfeeding. The good news is that you don't have to be as strict as during pregnancy when even small amounts of alcohol could harm your baby. But it still might be a good idea to avoid drinking this week while your baby has his second growth spurt because alcohol has been shown to interfere with how much milk he takes

Drinking while breastfeeding won't have any toxic effects on your baby since alcohol can't be stored in breast milk. Once you metabolise the alcohol, it is eliminated from your body and also from your milk. Having said that, small amounts of alcohol can be passed on to your baby if you feed him soon after drinking – alcohol levels in your milk peak after 30–90 minutes so wait an hour and a half per drink before nursing. This allows alcohol levels to fall. There's no need to express and throw your milk away unless your breasts become so engorged that you can't bear to wait to feed your baby.

The biggest problem with drinking and breastfeeding is that alcohol reduces levels of the breastfeeding hormone oxytocin, which triggers the 'let down' response that enables milk to travel to your nipple ready for your baby to drink. This can make it harder for your baby to suckle, and studies show that alcohol makes your baby nurse more frequently but consume less milk, which could lead to slower weight gain in the long term. As little as two units of alcohol (two small glasses of wine) is thought to interfere with how much milk your baby gets.

Bizarrely, drinking alcohol will actually make your breasts feel fuller. This is because it increases levels of the breastfeeding hormone prolactin, which stimulates the breasts to fill with milk. But this is no good to your baby because alcohol also affects 'let down' and suckling.

Bottle-feeding – teats

This week's growth spurt will mean a couple of very hungry days when your baby demands more food. Follow his lead and be prepared to feed him more frequently and to give him more in his bottle. You can also look at teat size this week as your baby may now want to guzzle hungrily so will need a faster teat with a bigger hole.

If his cheeks become sucked in with the effort of feeding, it means that the teat flow is too slow and you could try him on the next one up from newborn. Other signs that the hole in the teat is too small are if your baby takes a long time to finish his bottle or if he seems to almost give up rather than stop feeding because he's full. But if you give him a new teat and your baby splutters and seems to 'choke', then the milk flow is too fast and you'll need to revert back to a smaller one.

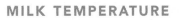

MILK TEMPERATURE

Up until now you'll have carefully warmed your baby's bottle to just the temperature he likes. You might want to think about gradually getting him used to cool milk now because this will be a lot more convenient, especially when you're out. If he's feeding well, try warming his bottles for slightly less time and see how he reacts. Once he's used to the cooler milk, cool it down a little more until you can do away with the warming process altogether.

NAPPIES

Number of wet nappies over 24 hours: 4–8
Number of dirty nappies over 24 hours: 0–6

You won't be changing as many nappies these days because as your baby grows he digests more of what he eats and so has fewer bowel movements. But there is a wide variation in how often babies poo – some will have several bowel movements a day, whereas others can have as few as one every four days, and sometimes babies become constipated.

Constipation

As long as your baby's stools are soft and he's not in pain when going to the toilet, it means that he isn't constipated. It's unusual for breastfed babies to become constipated because they have higher levels of a hormone called motilin, which assists the digestive system. But be aware that constipation does still affect some breastfed babies.

Bottle-fed babies are more likely to suffer from constipation because formula milk is more difficult to digest and poos will be thicker. Also formula milk doesn't contain any motilin to boost movement of the bowels.

Signs that your baby is constipated

If your baby's poos are soft there is no problem, even if he's straining. Look out for your baby having difficulty passing hard, dry-looking pellets, which means that he is constipated.

Treatment

Try massaging your baby's tummy gently in the bath to relieve tension – he'll be naked and relaxed in his warm bath making this an ideal time for a tummy massage. And if your baby is bottle-fed, check that you're making up his formula correctly and adding enough water because dehydration can cause constipation.

Speak to your health visitor about giving your baby a bottle of water (boiled and cooled) as this can sometimes relieve constipation. Prune juice can also help – but always speak to your health visitor. If your baby's constipation continues for more than 10 days, or if he seems uncomfortable, then see your doctor, who can prescribe laxatives and suppositories. NEVER use these without medical advice.

WASHING

For decades mothers have been sprinkling their infants with talc, giving them that delicious fresh baby smell. Using talc is one of the quickest ways to ensure that your baby's bottom is thoroughly dry after a nappy change, but think twice before using it.

Although talc is readily available in the baby sections of chemists and supermarkets, it has fallen out of favour with lots of mums who are wary of possible dangers. It turns out that there are indeed risks linked with using talc and that it's best avoided.

Firstly, lots of talcs are made with finely ground silicates – these particles are so small that they can be carried through the air and reach the lungs. Rarely, if a baby inhales talcum powder, it could lead to pneumonia, swelling of the airways and even death.

There has also been research into the possible link between talc and ovarian cancer. Talc can supposedly travel through the cervix and end up in the ovaries where it can cause irritation. But the evidence that talc causes ovarian cancer is inconclusive and dismissed by most experts. And there has been some concern that talc has a similar chemical structure to asbestos – but there isn't enough evidence to be able to draw similarities between the dangers of the two substances.

The best way to dry your baby's bottom is to expose the skin to the air, or use cotton wool, a face cloth, or even a hairdryer set on a low heat.

DEVELOPMENT AND PLAYING

Week six is smile week, when every parent excitedly waits for their baby to give them a big cheesy grin. Disappointingly, it doesn't happen quite like that – if you're lucky you'll get a tentative smirk while your baby makes eye contact with you. As you respond with big smiles of your own, your baby's smile will become more defined over the next few days. Those early smiling sessions with your baby are captivating and exciting, and certainly help make up for broken nights and hours of crying. You may only get one fleeting smile a day, but nearly all babies should engage and smile to some extent before they are seven weeks old.

Instead of recognising you by your outline, your baby now pays attention to your features, noticing your eyes, nose and mouth. This helps him to form a clearer memory of what you look like and not to be confused should you change your hairstyle or put glasses on. Being able to recognise faces in detail allows your baby to start recognising other people such as his dad, siblings and grandparents.

From around now your baby will enjoy watching things that move, so you could buy a mobile to hang above his changing table or cot. Black and white will be the easiest for your baby to see, but he will also be able to see some primary colours – bright colours are a better choice than pastels when it comes to choosing toys for your baby.

!SAFETY TIP OF THE WEEK!
Never give your baby aspirin

Aspirin can cause a rare condition called Reyes Syndrome in babies and children, which leads to liver damage and even death. So never give your baby aspirin. Infant paracetamol, such as Calpol, is the recommended painkiller for babies under six months. Breastfeeding mothers should also avoid aspirin.

WHEN TO SEE A DOCTOR

Umbilical granuloma

By now, your baby's cord stump will have dropped off and healed to an ordinary-looking belly button. However, in around one in 50 babies the cord drops off to reveal a bright red, sticky lump of tissue – this is called an umbilical granuloma. It contains no nerves so your baby doesn't feel a thing when it's touched and it should disappear within a few months.

If by now your baby doesn't have a regular-looking belly button you should get him checked by the doctor. Although an umbilical granuloma is nothing to worry about and probably won't even need treatment, in some cases the doctor gives it a helping hand by tying the tissue off with surgical thread so that it shrivels and drops off eventually, or it can be removed with silver nitrate. Both procedures are simple and painless.

WHAT'S HAPPENING TO MUM

If you're breastfeeding, then you'll notice around now that your breasts don't leak as much and that they seem softer. You might think that this is because you aren't making as much milk, but this isn't the case. What's happened is that your milk production has adjusted to your baby's demands.

Your womb will have shrunk to its pre-pregnant size as muscle fibres have now contracted. But your tummy will still be larger than pre-pregnancy because you have retained your pregnancy fat. This is nature's food store for your new baby and will gradually disappear as you breastfeed. It's too soon after the birth to diet, but you can resist indulging too much in chocolate, cake, biscuits and crisps, especially if you aren't breastfeeding. Don't be surprised if tiredness leaves you weak-willed as it's a biological fact that exhaustion makes you crave sugar and carbohydrates to keep energy levels up.

If you had a Caesarean, your wound should be fully healed by now and you can start lifting again. You can also start driving, but take it slowly because an emergency stop could hurt – check your insurance policy for the exact date that you can drive from.

PLANNING AHEAD
Booking your baby's immunisation appointment

Your baby should have his first immunisation (see page 133) at two months for diphtheria, tetanus, whooping cough, polio and *Haemophilus influenzae* Type B (Hib), plus another to protect against pneumococcal infection such as meningitis, septicaemia and pneumonia. Ask your health visitor whether you need to book your baby in at the clinic or with your GP, then make the appointment for the week after next. You will need to buy some Calpol (baby paracetamol), in case he gets a fever afterwards – check with your pharmacist that you have the version suitable for a two-month-old. Speak to your health visitor about any concerns you may have about giving your baby these vaccinations.

week 7

If you want to get your baby into a routine, this is about the earliest you can start thinking about it. Until now he has been too young to have any sort of timetable thrust upon him and has needed his cries for milk and cuddles to be met pretty much on demand.

It's still too soon to get your baby into a regimented feeding and sleeping regime, but what you can do is to gradually introduce a daily pattern. The advantage of a routine is that it will help you to recognise whether your baby is due for a feed or a sleep, which will take a lot of the guess work out of looking after him. This is particularly important from now onwards because hunger is no longer the main reason why your baby cries – he'll increasingly cry for other reasons such as tiredness and even boredom, making his needs ever more confusing.

A routine is by no means for everyone and plenty of mothers prefer to simply observe their baby's signals and respond instinctively to what he wants. The downside of a routine is that you can get so hung up on it that you overlook what your baby is telling you and you both end up miserable. There's even a risk of not feeding your baby enough if you're so preoccupied with sticking to a rigid timetable that you don't listen to his cries for milk.

A gentle routine, on the other hand, where you gradually encourage your baby into a feeding and sleeping pattern, should have advantages for both you and your baby. You'll spend less time offering him food when he's not hungry, and you're more likely to get him down to sleep before he becomes overtired and fractious. The result is that your baby will have his basic needs met quickly. The key, as always, is to respond to your baby and to stay sensitive to what he is telling you.

SLEEP

Total sleep required: 14–17 hours a day
Pattern: sleeps more at night than during the day – aim for daytime naps that total at least three hours

The textbook sleeping routine that many parents aim for is 12 hours of uninterrupted sleep at night and around two to three hours of napping during the day. A few babies adopt this sleep pattern by the time they are 16 weeks old, but many take up to a year or even longer. Taking some preparatory steps in these early weeks will certainly help to get your baby into a more organised sleep pattern later on.

Last week we talked about daytime napping and what to aim for (see page 112), but like most mums, you are no doubt more concerned about your baby's night-time sleeping habits. So it is night sleeping that we shall be focusing on over the next few weeks.

Sleeping for longer at night

Hopefully your baby is already sleeping for up to four or five hours during the night and sleeping more deeply as his body clock adapts to the concept of night-time. But if he still seems to have his days and nights confused then you'll need to address this as it's an essential step to getting him to sleep through the night and into a good routine.

Continue to keep things very low key at night with dim lighting and no playing (see page 81). During the day, don't let your baby nap for longer than three hours at a time – his total daytime napping shouldn't add up to more than about four hours.

One tried and tested method of helping your baby to sleep better at night is the old-fashioned ritual of taking your baby out in his pram for some fresh air during the day. This has now been backed by science, and a study published in the *Journal of Sleep Research* found that babies aged six, nine and twelve weeks old who were good night sleepers got double the amount of daylight between 12pm and 4pm as poor night sleepers. The researchers think this is because daylight exposure helps to regulate the sleep hormone melatonin which influences your baby's understanding of the difference between night and day.

CRYING

Number of hours your baby may cry in a day:
45 minutes–4.5 hours

Your baby's crying should begin to settle from this week and you'll notice a marked decline, albeit gradual, in his unexplained evening fussiness. Even colicky babies will soon show the first signs of improvement. This trend is set to continue for the next six weeks or so as your baby matures and feels less overwhelmed by the world.

FEEDING

Total milk required: 720–960 ml/24–32 oz a day
(up to 150 ml/5 oz per feed)
Pattern: 6–9 feeds a day

One big advantage of introducing a feeding routine is that you will have a pretty good idea when your baby is hungry and when he's crying from overtiredness. Another big plus to getting a feeding routine established is that you will find it easier in weeks to come to tweak it so that your baby eventually stops feeding at night, allowing you to get some much-longed-for sleep.

In week five (see page 102) we talked about gradually persuading your baby to wait longer between feeds as you attempt to get him to wait three hours from the start of one feed to the start of the next, and four hours at night. This week we continue this theme and look at more ways to help your baby to go for longer between feeds.

However desperate you are to establish a feeding pattern, always be guided by your baby – if he seems particularly hungry then he probably is, so feed him as much as he wants.

Breastfeeding

Establishing a feeding routine if you're breastfeeding will take longer than if you're bottle-feeding because your milk will have to adapt to the new feeding timetable, so allow a few weeks.

Begin by ensuring that your baby is getting enough rich hind milk (see page 102), and then for three days write down when he breast-feeds – chances are that you'll see a pattern emerge. The next step is to identify a 'disorganised' period in your baby's feeding schedule. Below are some of the most common disorganised periods which can occur each day, plus how to tackle them.

Morning snacking

Your baby may be having a few little feeds in the morning close together, say at 6.30am, 7am and 8.30am. This can occur if you wake up with engorged breasts and are tempted to give your baby a quick feed from both sides to relieve any discomfort. Your baby will miss out on the fatty hind milk and get hungry again very quickly. Try to feed him from one breast, and express a little milk from the other if you feel uncomfortable.

Afternoon indecision

You may find that your baby seems confused about what he wants at certain times of the day – perhaps in the afternoon he asks to be fed but doesn't seem particularly hungry. This usually happens because he's actually tired and needs to be put down for a sleep but feels overtired and thinks he needs comforting. Try feeding him plenty at the previous feed and then settle him before he becomes fractious.

Insatiable evening appetite

If your baby seems impossible to satisfy in the evenings and wants constant feeding, he's certainly not unusual. This generally happens because your milk supply is at its lowest at the end of the day when you are tired. You can try drinking plenty of fluids during the afternoon to keep your hydration levels up, and also relaxing in the late afternoon – getting hooked on a TV soap at about 5pm could work. Some mums express their excess milk in the morning and give this to their baby in the evening, and others give their baby a 'top-up' bottle of formula in the evening. Breastfeeding purists would argue against this because it upsets the natural balance between your baby's needs and your milk production – in most cases this symbiotic relationship resolves itself over the next few weeks and you will soon start to produce more milk in the evenings. But if you're desperate for a quick-fix solution then taking a few shortcuts won't upset the balance too much and plenty of mums swear by a bottle of formula at night as a way of keeping their baby going and getting a bit more sleep.

Night wakings you can set your clock by

You may find that you settle your baby for the night but then he wakes up an hour later demanding to be fed, or that you feed him at 2am only to be woken up at 3.30am every night without fail. Generally speaking, if your baby is waking up at the same time each night it is through habit rather than hunger. You can think about comforting your baby rather than feeding him if he's been fed within the last couple of hours, although if he's adamant that he's hungry then give in as he's still very young.

Bottle-feeding

It's easier to get your baby into a feeding routine if he's bottle-fed than if he is breastfed. This is partly because formula is digested more slowly so your baby can wait longer between feeds. But also because you can measure exactly how much milk he is taking.

If your baby has been gaining weight satisfactorily you can aim to feed him every three hours during the day from the start of one feed to the start of the next, and four hours at night (see page 102). For example, you may feed your baby at 7am, 10am, 1pm, 4pm, 7pm, 11pm, 3am, and again at 7am.

Add up how many ounces of milk your baby drinks in 24 hours, then divide this by seven to calculate how much you should give him per feed.

It will take your baby a few days to get used to his new schedule but he will gradually adapt, and once he does you'll find it much easier to anticipate his needs. Even following a schedule, your baby is bound to have times during the day or night when he is extra hungry, plus days when for some reason he wants to be fed more frequently. Try to remain sensitive to your baby's needs and to what he's telling you – he knows better than anyone exactly how much milk he should have.

LISTEN TO YOUR BABY

Just like adults, babies will have days when they're particularly hungry and need more milk. So it's important not to be too strict when it comes to following a feeding timetable and to always be led by your baby. Here's why:

- Your baby may be having a growth spurt and so need more milk.
- It could be a hot day, which makes him more thirsty.
- Perhaps he's feeling unwell, which can make him want lots of little feeds instead of a few big ones.
- If you're breastfeeding then you may be short of milk if you're tired, dehydrated or unwell, in which case your baby will demand extra feeds to compensate for the lack of milk.

NAPPIES

Number of wet nappies over 24 hours: 4–8
Number of dirty nappies over 24 hours: 0–6

Stool colours, what's normal?

Every parent worries about whether their baby's stools are normal, and most concerns turn out to be false alarms. Stools will vary a great deal in colour and pretty much any shade of brown or even green is considered healthy.

Green stools are more likely to occur if you are breastfeeding and your baby is getting too much fore milk and not enough hind milk. Fore milk is more dilute and contains more lactose, and it stimulates your baby's digestive tract to move milk along too quickly, producing green and often explosive stools. Don't worry if this is a one-off, but if your baby's weight gain is slow and he has consistently green stools, then be sure to feed him for long enough on one breast to allow him to get to the rich, fatty hind milk. You could also check with a breast-feeding counsellor that your baby is latching on correctly, enabling him to extract all the hind milk.

Occasionally green stools indicate a gut infection (see page 129).

You should also contact your doctor if your baby's stools are a creamy white colour or if they are black or red as this indicates blood in the stools (see page 130).

WASHING

Your baby may tremble when he becomes cool after a bath or if he is undressed. A quivering chin and jittery arms and legs are nothing to worry about – it's just a sign that your baby's nervous system is still underdeveloped. The trembling will stop over the next month or two.

DEVELOPMENT AND PLAYING

Your baby has reasonable head control and has lost the floppy fragility of the early days. If you use a sling, don't be tempted to turn your baby outwards to face the world. Lots of mums do this about now but it's too early – wait until your baby is three months old. At the moment he still doesn't have enough head control and is much happier curled up towards you, and his vision still isn't developed enough for him to enjoy looking around. Don't even think about putting your baby in a backpack-style carrier yet – you'll have to wait until he's at least six to eight months depending on his head control.

Your baby will still find faces (particularly yours) more interesting to look at than anything else. But he will also start to appreciate other visual stimuli. Any of the following will make his world more interesting: black and white photos of faces, chessboards, moving leaves, broad stripes and ceiling fans. Perhaps you could put his Moses basket under a tree in the garden on a warm day, or put a chessboard next to his changing table – he loves symmetrical patterns as they appear to swim before his eyes. It doesn't take much to entertain your baby at this age.

WHEN TO SEE A DOCTOR

Unusual stools

Babies' stools can be very varied and this is generally nothing to worry about (see page 127). But sometimes if you see something unusual, you should contact your doctor. Here's a checklist of what to look out for:

White

Always see a doctor if your baby's stools are creamy white as this indicates a possible liver problem. This can be serious so you need to see your doctor quickly, and if possible, take a small stool sample with you. White stools are full of fat that hasn't been absorbed in the gut, and they also float – obviously difficult to detect as your baby is still in nappies.

Green

The only time you need to worry about green stools is if your baby also has a fever (temperature above 38°C/100.4°F), and if he is vomiting or seems unwell as this indicates a gut infection. Again, take your baby to your doctor quickly as he may become dehydrated.

It's also common for babies to get very mild gut infections which result in green stools without feeling unwell. These infections often go unnoticed, so if your baby seems okay in himself then there's no need to worry about the occasional green stool. Other reasons for green stools are if your baby is on medication, if you're breastfeeding and taking iron supplements or if he is sensitive to something in your diet such as dairy products – in this case he could have other symptoms such as eczema. If you suspect this then go and see your GP and ask for a referral to a dietitian.

Red or black

A red or black colour can indicate blood in your baby's stools which can be alarming, although the cause usually turns out to be something quite innocent such as cracked nipples (see below). But you should always report the problem to your health visitor and to your doctor if your baby seems unwell, because blood in the stools can sometimes indicate a serious condition.

A common cause of blood in the stools is if you are breastfeeding and you have cracked nipples – as your baby sucks he can easily suck quite a lot of blood too. This isn't anything to worry about and the blood won't do your baby any harm.

These stools may appear black because the blood was ingested by your baby and is converted in his bowel, changing from bright red to black. Another reason for black stools is if your baby has been prescribed iron supplements.

Stools may have bright red blood in them if your baby has an anal fissure (tear) which can happen if he's been constipated. You won't be able to see the tear yourself, but the blood will be bright red and will coat the stool. Fissures usually heal by themselves but you should try to prevent your baby becoming constipated (see page 116).

If your baby has diarrhoea he may have blood in his stools because he has a bowel infection and his gut wall may be damaged. He will already seem very unwell if this is the case and should definitely see a doctor if he hasn't already done so.

WHAT'S HAPPENING TO MUM

A particularly distressing birth can leave you feeling traumatised and you may find that you're still telling everyone about it as you re-live the gory details. You might be vowing never to have another baby because you couldn't put yourself through the birth nightmare again, even though your original plan was to have four kids. If your birth memories are still vivid and you really can't move on, contact your hospital midwife team and ask for an appointment to talk it through.

You can also write to your director of midwifery asking for a copy of your hospital records and birthing notes. Women often find it reassuring when they understand exactly why procedures such as an episiotomy or emergency Caesarean were carried out. You won't be the first woman who has wanted to talk about her birth to a professional, and you should get a very sympathetic response.

PLANNING AHEAD
Child Benefit

If you haven't yet sorted out Child Benefit, make sure that you do so soon because you will lose money if you delay. If neither you or your partner earn more than £60,000 your child will be entitled to some benefits, and if neither of you earn more than £50,000 your child will be entitled to the full amount – £20.30 for the first child and £13.40 for each additional child.

Child Benefit can be backdated for up to three months, so you need to apply in the next few weeks to ensure that you don't miss any payments. You will need to send your child's birth certificate (which you now have as you've registered your child) plus an application form to the Inland Revenue.

You may have got an application form in your Bounty Pack (given to new mothers in hospital) or you can contact the Inland Revenue on 0845 302 1444, or go to www.hmrc.gov.uk/childbenefit.

Child Tax Credit

You will be entitled to a tax rebate if your joint income with your partner is £66,000 or less – or if you alone earn less than £66,000 and you are single. For more information contact the Inland Revenue on 0844 496 6507 or go to www.hmrc.gov.uk/TAXCREDITS.

week 8

Your baby should hopefully be booked in for his immunisations this week, which may make you feel a little apprehensive. It's normal for mums to worry about whether the vaccine is safe, and how their baby will cope with having injections. As far as safety and side effects are concerned, the first year of your child's vaccination programme isn't particularly controversial and pretty much all babies are immunised around this age.

There are two injections which are usually given in each of your baby's thighs – firstly the five-in-one jab protects against diphtheria, tetanus, whooping cough, polio, and *Haemophilus influenzae* Type B (Hib) – an infection that can cause pneumonia and a particular strain of meningitis. And the other injection is for pneumococcal infection, which can cause meningitis, pneumonia, septicaemia and ear infections. At three months your baby will be given a booster five-in-one jab, plus another for meningitis C. Then at four months he'll have three jabs: his third and final five-in-one jab, as well as another meningitis C jab, and another pneumococcal jab. After this your baby won't have any more jabs until he is 12 months old when he'll get his final meningitis C booster, as well as a Hib booster.

The jabs will protect your baby against a long list of killer diseases at just about the time when his immunity is starting to decline – all babies are born with quite a lot of immunity that they get from their mothers while in the womb.

In the past there have been some scare stories linked with the vaccine but these concerns are no longer an issue. Firstly, there was some anxiety that the vaccines contained a mercury-based preservative called thiomersal, but the new vaccines no longer use this preservative. Another worry was that the live oral polio vaccine had a tiny risk of paralysis, but now a new vaccine has been introduced that is inactivated – not live – so has no risk whatsoever of causing paralysis. The polio vaccine is no longer administered orally but is given as an injection and is part of the five-in-one vaccine.

Finally the whooping cough vaccine received bad press in the early 1970s when it was said to cause fits, but this research turned out to be flawed and there is no proven link. And the whooping cough vaccine has now been updated and contains less toxins and also has fewer side effects such as swelling and redness.

You may be worried about how your baby will respond to having needles jabbed into his thighs. Most two-month-olds barely notice their first thigh being injected but often get upset when their second thigh is jabbed a couple of minutes later, probably because they cotton on to what's happening. If you breastfeed, try feeding your baby while he's being vaccinated, as this can sometimes help. Otherwise just give him a big cuddle afterwards and he'll calm down within seconds.

If your baby has a fever, you should postpone his immunisation appointment for another week. The nurse won't mind at all, and probably wouldn't do the vaccination even if you did turn up as your baby could end up feeling quite unwell. And also the vaccine won't be as effective because your baby's immune system will already be working hard so won't be able to kick in as vigorously to attack the vaccine. This means that not as much resistance can be built up. But if he's got a cold and no fever then it's fine to go ahead with the immunisation. Finally, if your baby has ever had any sort of fit then you should tell the doctor or nurse who is giving the injection.

Your baby will probably feel unwell for a day or so after his vaccination (see page 142) but should then be absolutely fine.

SLEEP

Total sleep required: 14–17 hours a day
Pattern: sleeps more at night than during the day – aim for your baby to have at least five hours of uninterrupted sleep at night, plus daytime naps that total at least three hours

Half of all babies will now sleep for five hours or more at night. If your baby does this, then congratulations – there are a lot of parents out there who are still struggling by on no more than three hours of unbroken sleep a night. If your baby doesn't yet have a big night-sleep, then take heart because the odds do improve – 70 per cent of all three-month-old babies go for at least five hours at night. But in the meantime, have another look at the golden rule of sleep training, which is to put your baby down awake (see page 66).

Babies, like adults, drift in and out of sleep throughout the night, waking up several times. Your job is to teach your baby to drift back off to sleep again, all by himself, so that eventually he doesn't need rocking or even feeding. Once he can self-soothe, you will be closer to that elusive but all-important goal of him sleeping through the night.

The more practice your baby has at getting himself off to sleep in these early days, the easier things will be in a couple of months when you're teaching him to sleep through the night. So do allow time each day to teach your baby to self-soothe, even if it feels as though he's not making progress. This skill is essential to sleeping through the night and your baby will eventually learn. If you haven't had much luck with the self-soothe technique yet, it could be for one of the following reasons:

1. He falls asleep during feeds

This is very common and needs to be resolved in the next few weeks before your baby becomes too set in his ways (which generally happens after three months).

Once you are sure your baby has had enough milk and is just hanging on for comfort, gently pull the teat or nipple away to encourage him to go to sleep without the comfort of sucking. What's quite likely to happen is that your baby will become suddenly alert and complain, in which case give him back the breast or bottle and try again next time. You may have to try 100 times before he remains calm enough to fall asleep without being fed – but put the effort in now and you will reap the rewards in weeks to come when your baby is able to fall asleep without being nursed.

2. You are putting your baby down when he is still too alert

Wait until your baby is dopey and relaxed before putting him in his cot. It might seem like cheating to wait until he's half asleep, but bear in mind that your baby is learning quite a difficult skill and needs all the help you can give him.

3. You aren't giving your baby enough time to settle himself

It can take a few minutes for babies to settle themselves so don't rush in too quickly – a little bit of grizzling and moaning can be a sign that your baby is about to nod off, so don't be too hasty to pick him up again. But if you're sure that it's not going to work then pick him up and start again.

WHEN TO FORGET ABOUT SLEEP TRAINING

There will be times when it's easy to put your baby down awake and settle him quickly. But at other times he'll need more help getting to sleep, which is when you can resort to the rocking technique that you've perfected over the weeks. Although the ultimate aim is self-soothing, you can forget trying to teach your baby anything if he's ill, overtired, has wind, or perhaps he's just drifted off and the phone wakes him – he'll be upset and a bit of help getting him to sleep again could save you both quite a lot of anguish. The more often your baby goes off to sleep by himself the better. So aim over the next few months to minimise the help you give him going to sleep and maximise the number of times he gets to sleep by himself.

CRYING

Number of hours your baby may cry in a day:
40 minutes–4 hours

Your baby will continue to cry less this week, and now it's time to start thinking about when it's okay to let him cry. For some unknown reason, it's very common for babies to cry a bit before they go off to sleep. So if you are teaching your baby to self-soothe himself to sleep, as mentioned above, listen carefully so that you can start to recognise this pre-sleep grizzling. Once you know this cry, you won't rush to 'help' when your baby is about to drop off. Don't let his cry become a distressed howl because your baby is still too young to cry himself to sleep, but a bit of gentle grizzling is fine. The other benefit of learning to recognise the 'going to sleep grizzle' is that over the next few months when your baby wakes in the night and doesn't need food but just a few moments to re-settle himself, you'll know not to rush in.

FEEDING

Total milk required: 720–960 ml/24–32 oz a day
(up to 180 ml/6 oz per feed)
Pattern: 6–9 feeds a day

By now you're better at understanding your baby and recognising if he feels uncomfortable after a feed. It's very common for parents to suspect milk intolerance or an allergy when their baby is about two months old, but it rarely turns out to be the case as these only affect around one in 50 to 100 babies and are more common in bottle-fed babies. If your baby does in fact become allergic or intolerant to cows' milk, he'll probably grow out of it by the time he is one, and nearly all babies grow out of it by the age of two.

So although it would be nice to have something specific to blame for your baby's never-ending grizzling and indigestion, the reality is that babies often cry for unspecific reasons and you'll probably never know why. In the meantime it's important not to put your baby on to a special hypoallergenic milk formula unnecessarily, or without medical supervision, because these special milks are inferior to cows' milk formulas, which are closer to breast milk.

If you are breastfeeding, don't cut out dairy products unnecessarily because pregnancy would have left your calcium stores depleted and you should be eating more dairy than ever (see page 143).

Signs that your baby is allergic to milk

A true allergy is quite dramatic and your baby will be sick several times a day, have watery poos (perhaps even blood stained) and poor weight gain. He may also get eczema or a rash, and a runny nose. It's more likely that your baby has a milk allergy if either you or his father also suffer from milk allergy, or any other allergy, including being atopic, i.e. having eczema, asthma or hayfever.

Signs that your baby is intolerant to milk

An intolerance will just make your baby sick occasionally, and have slightly runny poos which may be mucous. He may also suffer from painful indigestion.

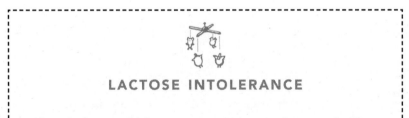

LACTOSE INTOLERANCE

Your baby could become sensitive to lactose (milk sugar) after a bout of gastroenteritis and he may suffer from stomach cramps, wind and even frothy poos for a couple of weeks while his gut learns to cope with lactose again. But your baby is extremely unlikely to be lactose intolerant for any other reason as this generally only affects adults and older children. It happens when you don't have the enzyme to break down lactose, but all babies have this enzyme.

Breastfeeding

Only a particularly sensitive baby would be affected by cows' milk protein in your breast milk, so it's unlikely that you need to eliminate dairy products from your diet. If you decide to go ahead though, do so for two weeks and there should be a noticeable improvement of your baby's symptoms if there's an underlying problem. Otherwise he's obviously not intolerant or allergic to cows' milk and you can eat and drink dairy products again. If, however, you do suspect he has a problem with dairy foods, then speak to your health visitor or GP as this will affect your baby when he starts on solids.

Bottle-feeding

If your doctor confirms that your baby is intolerant or allergic to milk, then changing your baby's formula is a quick-fix solution. There's a formula called hydrolysate in which the milk protein is pre-digested – this is available on prescription only. If symptoms disappear, then under your doctor's supervision you will probably be advised to reintroduce cows' milk-based formula to your baby, then if symptoms reappear you can be pretty sure of the diagnosis. Some babies are also put on soya milk, but the problem with this is that soya allergies or intolerances can also occur so there may be no improvement of symptoms.

NAPPIES

Number of wet nappies over 24 hours: 4–8
Number of dirty nappies over 24 hours: 0–5

You may have noticed that your baby's stools are on the loose side, possibly bordering on looking like diarrhoea. But runny stools are normal for babies, particularly if they are breastfed. However, if your baby gets true diarrhoea, this needs to be treated quickly to prevent dehydration.

When not to worry

The occasional explosive nappy that leaks up your baby's back isn't a worry, unless of course he seems unwell or has a fever. Explosive poos may occur in a breastfed baby because he is drinking too much lactose-rich fore milk. This is dilute and stimulates the digestive tract to move things along too fast resulting in explosive poos. Try waiting longer for your baby to finish one breast before moving him to the other – think one breast per feed, and only swap him over if he is definitely still hungry.

When to worry

If your baby's stools are noticeably looser, there is an excessive amount, and they are explosive, much smellier, more watery, and more frequent, then this indicates diarrhoea. The big danger with diarrhoea is dehydration so feed your baby more frequently than usual and see your health visitor or doctor within 24 hours if symptoms continue.

WASHING

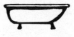

The big bath

You can put your baby into the big bath this week, if you haven't done so already. He may be getting quite big for his baby bath and be wriggling around so much that he's making quite a splash. If you've had the small bath on a bath stand, it's definitely time to move it to the floor in case it topples over. It's worth getting a rubber bathmat for the big bath to stop him slipping, and even a specially designed baby bath seat, which will make hair washing a lot easier.

DEVELOPMENT AND PLAYING

This week your baby may start to make consonant sounds, so listen out for him saying, 'Goo, gaa, coo', and so on. Copy his sounds and he'll 'talk' back to you.

Your baby will open his hand more often as he loses his grasp reflex. Instead of clutching indiscriminately at anything you put in his fist, he'll actually grasp for objects more purposefully for a few seconds and begin to reach out and slap at things in front of him. So you could lie him under a baby gym or put a string of beads or toys above his cot or pram that he can enjoy trying to bash.

If your baby still isn't smiling at all, then see your doctor. It's possible that he has a developmental problem or that he has a visual impairment that means he's not responding to faces.

!SAFETY TIP OF THE WEEK!
Remove strings and ribbons

Always remove string or ribbons which are longer than 10 cm/4 in from your baby's toys to avoid strangulation. You should also avoid using strings and ribbons on dummies and clothes.

WHEN TO SEE A DOCTOR

Vaccination reactions

The most likely reaction your baby will have is to cry briefly when he's given his jabs and then be grizzly for up to 48 hours after his vaccination – it's normal to feel unwell. You can alleviate this by giving him infant paracetamol, such as Calpol, 20 minutes after his vaccination and then every four hours or more if necessary – make sure you read the dosage instructions carefully though.

It's better to give Calpol routinely after his jab rather than wait for symptoms as this will prevent your baby from feeling poorly. And it's okay to give your baby Calpol even though he's just two months old if it's to alleviate the effects of his routine jabs.

A slight fever, up to 38ºC/100.4ºF, is nothing to worry about – just avoid wrapping your baby up in too many layers of clothing or bedding and keep him well hydrated. There might be a small lump at the injection site, which can last a couple of weeks – this can be a little tender so be careful when dressing and bathing your baby.

A known but rare side effect of the vaccination is that babies can have a fit, causing uncontrolled rhythmical movements, eye rolling, lip smacking, staring, and/or unconsciousness. Vaccine-related fits occur within 48 hours and are not a serious problem – just very distressing for parents. If this happens, call an ambulance, put your baby in the recovery position on his side to keep his airway free, and time how many seconds the fit lasts (the doctors will ask you this). You can also cool your baby down if he feels hot – remove his clothes and dab him with tepid water. It is essential that your baby is seen by a doctor because other causes of fits can be a lot more serious, for example meningitis or epilepsy, and these need to be ruled out.

Very few babies get fits though, and some won't even feel unwell following their jabs. So if nothing happens to your baby in the first 48 hours, you can stop worrying. Very rarely, babies turn out to have an extreme allergic reaction to a vaccine and can go into anaphylactic shock, where they have breathing difficulties and collapse. This only occurs in one child per 500,000 and will happen almost immediately while you're still at the surgery – your doctor will know how to treat it.

WHAT'S HAPPENING TO MUM

During pregnancy, calcium from your body is passed to your baby for his bones and teeth, and you may lose more if you are breastfeeding.

So make sure that you are eating a calcium-rich diet. A pint of milk provides your daily quota, as does a big lump of cheese, or two-and-a-half yoghurts. While green vegetables also provide calcium, you have to eat unrealistic amounts to get enough – six portions of spinach or 22 portions of broccoli a day. So if you're not a big fan of dairy products, it's worth thinking about taking a calcium supplement.

Long term, breastfeeding has a positive effect on your bones and the lost bone mass of nursing mums is restored within a year of stopping breastfeeding. It's also been shown that the longer you breastfeed the lower your risk of osteoporosis.

PLANNING AHEAD
Buy a cot

It's time to think about buying a cot because your baby is not only getting bigger and taking up more space in his Moses basket, but he is also kicking a lot and becoming increasingly likely to topple it over. Cots can take up to a couple of weeks to be delivered so start shopping now. It's okay to use a sturdy second-hand cot, but buy a new mattress to reduce the risk of cot death. When buying a cot, consider the following: whether it can be converted into a toddler bed, whether the sides are high enough to prevent a two-year-old climbing out and how solid it is – a strong toddler will happily shake and rock a flimsy cot across a room.

week 9

If you want Child Benefit back payments to be made from the day your baby was born the deadline is this week. If you don't send off your form in the next few days you could lose money, as Child Benefit can't be backdated by more than three months (see page 131).

Hopefully by now you'll be feeling as though you have come out of the newborn fog. Your baby will be smiley and responsive, slightly easier to look after now that he cries a little less, needs fewer feeds and nappy changes, and hopefully sleeps a little longer at night.

If you've got a particularly fussy baby or if he's colicky then your evenings will still seem pretty dismal, but things really are about to change. Improvements will be very gradual but your baby is now over two months old and vastly different to when he was first born. So hang on in there if things are still tricky because it's all going to get easier very soon if it hasn't done so far.

SLEEP

Total sleep required: 14–16 hours a day
Pattern: sleeps more at night than during the day – aim for
your baby to have at least five hours of uninterrupted sleep at
night, plus daytime naps that total at least three hours

You will almost certainly be able to soothe your baby more skilfully than when he was first born as you know exactly how to hold him, whether he likes sshing or singing, and his favourite rocking rhythm. But while it's extremely useful to be able to get your baby off to sleep quickly it's also important that he learns to self-soothe (see page 135).

One problem with becoming too proficient at settling your baby is that he can get hooked on an elaborate settling ritual and refuse to go to sleep any other way. Perhaps you have to rock him quite vigorously in his buggy to get him off, or dance around the bedroom singing, or even walk up and down the stairs. While you've discovered what seems to be your baby's 'off switch', there's a fine line between being able to get your baby off to sleep and letting him get into bad habits that will have to be undone at some time in the future. Being aware that such habits are becoming established will help you stop them from becoming too ingrained. You don't have to do anything drastic, just gradually tone things down a bit – it takes babies about three days to get used to new patterns.

Your ultimate aim is to be able to put your baby in his cot then walk out of the room and leave him to fall asleep by himself. Avoiding complex settling rituals is a step towards this goal. So, if at the moment you rock the buggy vigorously, try rocking it more gently – it may take your baby longer to settle at first, but he'll soon get used to it. Gradually you can try not rocking it at all. Or if you dance around the bedroom singing, try cutting out the singing (you can continue dancing with him for now). Again it will take your baby a little longer to settle because he's become used to your singing, but he'll soon learn to live without it, even if he protests for a while. The next step is to slow the dancing to a gentle rocking, which may take a few days for your baby to get used to.

The worst habit parents get into is driving their baby around in the car – if you do this then stop now. Yes, your baby will howl the place down, but if you make sure that he is fed, has a clean nappy and is safely in your arms, or in his cot with a reassuring hand on his tummy, you can be confident that he doesn't have any real problems. The next step is to wait it out, which can take perhaps an hour if he's become very used to the car, although at this age it will be more likely to take 20 minutes. Do this for three to four nights and you'll break the habit and your baby will be happy to go to sleep in your arms, or in his cot – whichever you choose. This won't be easy to achieve, but the alternative is to drive your baby round every night until he's four or older – plenty of parents end up in this predicament. It's much easier to break bad habits now than when your baby is older than three months as he will become more difficult to re-programme. Although it can seem tedious teaching your baby to get to sleep with less help from you, if you put the time in now you'll save hours of tedium in the future.

CRYING

Number of hours your baby may cry in a day:
30 minutes–3.5 hours

The amount of time your baby cries continues to decrease this week, and if your baby has colic then you can look forward to a dramatic improvement in his crying in just a few weeks. Last week we talked about how you can start to deliberately leave your baby for a couple of minutes when he cries in the night to see if he re-settles himself (see page 137). You may also want to start leaving him for a few moments during the day without rushing to pick him up – for example if he starts crying while you're getting dressed or having a shower. Just keep talking to him, give yourself permission to continue with what you are doing rather than rushing over to your baby; hopefully, when he sees that you are relaxed he'll feel a little more secure himself.

FEEDING

Total milk required: 720–960 ml/24–32 oz a day (up to 210 ml/7 oz per feed)
Pattern: 6–9 feeds a day

If you've got a fussy baby or one who suffers from colic then you're probably desperate to find a way to settle him. You are bound to explore countless reasons why he grizzles so much as you search for a quick solution. Allergies and intolerances are often blamed (see page 138). Or if your baby drinks formula then you've no doubt wondered whether switching to another brand might soothe his indigestion. However, it's unlikely that changing your diet or switching formula will make any difference whatsoever. Frustratingly, it's a case of accepting that it's perfectly normal for some babies to be very fussy and to cry a lot for the first three months.

Breastfeeding

If you breastfeed, you may have been told by well-meaning relatives and friends to stop eating chocolate, coffee, spicy foods, pulses, cheese and countless other foods because they can affect your milk and cause your baby wind and indigestion. It turns out that this is nonsense and you can eat more or less what you like when you breastfeed.

It's true that cabbage, beans and broccoli may make you windy, but this wind is contained in your gut not your blood, and breast milk is made from what passes into your blood. So your baby won't become any windier when you eat these foods. As for garlic upsetting your baby, again this isn't the case. Garlic does affect the flavour of your milk but studies have shown that it doesn't affect your baby's digestion. And babies in other cultures don't have any more colic even if their mothers eat dishes packed with garlic and hot spices. So if your baby seems windy after you've eaten a spicy bean curry it is almost certainly a coincidence. After all, babies fuss constantly and it's tempting to point the finger at something you've eaten recently as this gives you a sense of control. But young babies often cry for unexplained reasons and for the moment there are no quick-fix solutions.

Caffeine has been linked with feeding problems and wakefulness, but this won't happen if you only drink a few cups of coffee a day because very little caffeine actually passes into your milk. The ideal intake, recommended by paediatricians, is one to three cups a day. Chocolate also contains caffeine, which is why some people will tell you not to eat it while breastfeeding, but you'd have to eat vast quantities to affect your baby.

There is always a chance that your baby has a genuine allergy or intolerance to a particular food in which case he will be affected by your diet (see page 140). But the likelihood of this is slim – the most common offender is cows' milk and only 1 to 2 per cent of babies are affected. It's even more unusual for other foods to affect your baby so there's little point in trying to eliminate any foods from your diet.

If you're truly convinced that a particular food is causing your baby problems, then cut it out for a couple of weeks to see if there is any improvement. When you re-introduce the offending food, bear in mind that what you eat affects your milk within four to six hours.

Why you should eat healthily while breastfeeding

Despite what you might think, a healthy diet won't make your milk any more nutritious than if you eat lots of junk food – your baby will still get all the nutrients he needs, including iron and calcium. The only loser will be you because you'll go short of important vitamins and minerals and feel run-down. So the real reason you should eat a healthy diet when breastfeeding is to keep yourself healthy and your energy levels high. Another good reason to eat lots of fruit and vegetables is that your diet affects the flavour of your milk. Scientists have found that when babies are weaned on to solids they are more likely to enjoy fruit and vegetables if their breastfeeding mother included these in her diet.

Bottle-feeding

You may have heard of mums who switched formula and noticed vast improvements in the amount their baby cried, but the change in formula is unlikely to have been the reason. Babies will suddenly be less fussy about having wind as they get older, this usually happens when they are about three months old. But still lots of mums long to find a magic answer. Of course you can try different formulas, or even switch from a powder to a liquid version of the same brand, but the only real difference is in the taste and your baby may prefer some brands to others.

Don't be tempted by low-iron formulas as there is no evidence that these reduce your baby's wind, despite the claims that they can help colic, wind and discomfort. Low-iron formula milk contains insufficient iron for your baby, while regular formula milk contains high amounts because the iron isn't as easily absorbed from formula milk as it is from breast milk.

Unless your baby is definitely allergic or intolerant to cows' milk, there is no point in switching to another formula. You will be better off ensuring that your baby is winded properly halfway through his feed, and that he doesn't suck in too much air when feeding – ensure that his mouth is open wide with his lips tightly round the teat.

NAPPIES

Number of wet nappies over 24 hours: 4–8
Number of dirty nappies over 24 hours: 0–5

If you use disposable nappies, you've probably had the occasional pang of guilt as you think about landfill sites – your baby alone will use over 5,000 nappies from now until he is potty trained, and these will take at least a couple of hundred years to decompose. But if you've not given the environment too much consideration so far, then you might want to around now because your baby is becoming a little easier to look after.

Before you switch to reusable nappies, however, there are a few points to consider. Firstly, these aren't as ecologically friendly as you'd expect because it takes energy to wash and dry them and then there's the issue of soap run-off and water use. On balance they are probably better for the environment because there isn't the problem of decomposing. But their big downside is the inconvenience of having the extra laundry, carrying dirty nappies home with you when you've been out with your baby, and dealing with more leaks as these nappies aren't as efficient as disposables. Some people argue that reusables are better for nappy rash because your baby only has pure cotton next to his skin rather than synthetic disposables. Although others say that disposables whisk away moisture more efficiently making them better for nappy rash. The big plus with washable nappies is the cost because, although there's an initial outlay when you buy around 18 nappies, it works out cheaper in the long run than disposables. You'll probably save about £500 over the next couple of years if you swap to cloth nappies.

If you decide to try reusable nappies then you could consider a laundry service that delivers nappies to your door once a week and takes away the soiled ones. The nappies are washed at higher temperatures than you'd use at home, which helps reduce your baby's risk of nappy rash as all harmful bacteria are killed. Some local authorities are encouraging parents to make this swap by offering cash incentives of up to £80 towards the cost of buying the cloth nappies in the first place, plus laundry bills. Speak to your health visitor about subsidies in your area if you're interested.

For your nearest laundry service try www.goreal.org.uk. Just enter your postcode for your nearest nappy agent who will come to your home and talk you through the various non-disposable options and may even offer a free initial trial.

WASHING

Until now you may have been using olive oil to moisturise your baby's skin. After a couple of months it's quite common for a baby's skin to become a bit dry so you might want to take other measures to keep it moisturised. Avoid using bubble bath as this contains detergent, which is drying. Shampoo is also drying so limit hair washing to once a week – babies and children don't need constant scrubbing and cleaning. Instead of using soap, you can use something called Aqueous Cream to clean your baby. This is available from chemists in large plastic tubs and can also be used to moisturise your baby's skin after the bath. It doesn't have the nice scent of the prettily packaged cosmetic baby moisturisers, and it isn't absorbed so easily as it is very thick. But although less pleasant to use, Aqueous Cream is recommended by doctors for babies who have dry or sensitive skin because it is effective in locking in moisture, and also it's cheap and fragrance free.

DEVELOPMENT AND PLAYING

Your baby will be less curled up when you put him on his tummy and will be able to lift his head for about 10 seconds or longer. Encourage this by putting brightly coloured toys in front of him. As your baby continues to learn how to use his hands he will start to enjoy rattles or anything that makes a noise. He's also old enough to start making a link between what he's doing with his hands and what he hears and sees, which is why noisy, brightly coloured plastic toys are popular from around this age.

It still takes a few seconds for your baby to focus on an object, as you'll observe if you hold a toy in front of your baby – he'll stare blankly and blink before really seeing the object.

!SAFETY TIP OF THE WEEK!
Don't leave your baby to fall

Your baby is old enough to be propped up on the sofa surrounded by cushions, but only do this if you are sitting with him. Never leave your baby unattended on the sofa, for example while you whiz across the room to grab the TV controls, because every year babies break their bones from falling off furniture before they are even a year old.

WHEN TO SEE A DOCTOR

Eczema

Eczema commonly develops when your baby is two months old, so if your baby's going to get it you may see the first signs around now. About one in seven babies suffer from eczema, and if you or your baby's father have eczema, hayfever or asthma then his chance of eczema increases to almost one in three because the condition is hereditary. Although there isn't a cure for eczema, the condition can be managed and generally it doesn't become too serious. In a lot of cases it clears up entirely by the time your child is two, and will almost certainly improve and hopefully disappear by the time he is a teenager.

Look out for dry, scaly skin on your baby's cheeks, and behind his knees and elbows – although eczema can appear anywhere on his body. Another way to detect eczema is to note that affected areas will feel rough to touch, as though covered in an invisible layer of fine sand. The problems don't really begin until eczema flares up and then it becomes extremely itchy and you'll probably see red spots that blister and weep clear fluid. Your baby will scratch, sometimes until his skin bleeds, and then there is a risk of infection. As soon as you suspect eczema get the diagnosis confirmed by your GP, who will write you a prescription for an emollient to put on your baby's skin up to six times a day, plus Oilatum – an oil to add to the bath which helps moisturise the skin, and a mild steroid cream to control the flare-ups. Do go back to your doctor when supplies of creams and eczema bath products run low as children's prescriptions are free and these products will get costly over the months.

What you can do at home

It's important to treat your baby's eczema every day, even between flare-ups when it's not causing him problems. Keeping your baby's skin well hydrated will help strengthen it and reduce the severity of flare-ups, so always add Oilatum to his bath, then smother him with an emollient once you've dried him. If you don't get on with the emollient you've been prescribed, try a different one as there are lots on the market and it's worth experimenting until you find something that you like using – 50/50 White Soft Paraffin is popular with parents of extreme eczema sufferers.

Only wash your baby's hair once a week, using fragrance-free shampoo for babies with sensitive skin, and instead of soap use an Aqueous Cream to clean your baby (see page 152). You can also keep your baby's nails short and put him in scratch mittens at night to reduce the damage he does when his eczema itches. And dress him in cotton clothes that let the skin breathe and keep it cool – you can buy seamless baby clothes to minimise irritation from www.eczemaclothing.com.

It's also worth investigating whether your child has a milk intolerance (see page 139) as this affects up to 1 per cent of babies. But speak to your doctor about this as you shouldn't alter your baby's diet without medical supervision. When your baby's eczema flares up, apply steroid cream immediately, up to three times a day or as directed. Don't delay using the steroid cream in the hope that the eczema will calm down – it probably won't and using the steroid cream quickly could prevent the flare-up from becoming too serious. While steroid creams can cause the skin to thin if used long term, using them for a couple of weeks during a flare-up is fine because these creams are mild and contain no more than 1 per cent steroid. So be liberal and let them do their job. You can be more sparing on your baby's face because the skin is more sensitive – your doctor may even prescribe a milder steroid cream for the face. And you should be particularly careful around the eye 'bag' area as the skin is extremely thin here – some doctors say that you shouldn't apply any steroid here at all so do discuss this with your GP.

What your doctor can do

Although baby eczema is usually quite mild, and is never life-threatening, a bad case can be extremely distressing. It can keep your baby awake at night as he scratches his skin raw and cries, which in turn keeps the whole family up. Coupled with the fact that severe eczema can be disfiguring, particularly on the face, this condition is upsetting to cope with as a parent and requires a lot of time and effort to treat it. As well as seeing your doctor for the initial diagnoses and getting regular checks and repeat prescriptions, you must also get medical help if the eczema weeps and bleeds because there is a risk of secondary infection. Your doctor may prescribe a topical antibiotic cream or perhaps oral antibiotics in severe cases. If the eczema is causing your child particular distress then you may need to wrap him in specially designed moisturised bandages at night, and perhaps speak to your doctor about giving your baby an antihistamine – this has an anti-itch effect as well as being a sedative.

BEWARE OF ALTERNATIVE TREATMENTS

Eczema is a distressing condition with no cure and this creates a desperation often exploited by charlatans. It's also a condition that clears up spontaneously, which is why many unqualified gurus and unlicensed products claim to cure the condition.

If you decide to explore the alternative route, you could end up wasting your money and make the condition worse because many alternative products don't have a licence and haven't been tested. Also the gurus who claim to treat eczema may try to dissuade you from using conventional treatments prescribed by your GP. But this would be extremely dangerous should your baby's eczema become infected.

By all means try a more 'natural' emollient on your baby's skin if someone you know swears by it, just patch test it first and wait 48 hours. But bear in mind that if it was really that effective then GPs and paediatricians up and down the country would be recommending it to their patients because they routinely treat children with extreme eczema and are as keen as any parent to find a cure.

WHAT'S HAPPENING TO MUM

It takes up to two years for your iron stores to return to pre-pregnancy levels, so make sure that you're having plenty of this vital nutrient. Good sources of iron include red meat, dried apricots, dark green vegetables, eggs and fortified breakfast cereal. Drink orange juice with your iron because vitamin C increases absorption, and cut back on tea as tannin inhibits absorption. If you think that you might be anaemic then speak to your doctor about taking an iron supplement – signs of anaemia include your lower eyelids being pale pink instead of bright red, and feeling tired and sometimes breathless. You could also take an iron tonic, which is less likely to cause constipation than a supplement.

During this week you may well be contacted by someone from the health visiting team to carry out an assessment of whether you are suffering from post-natal depression (PND). You'll be given the Edinburgh questionnaire to fill in. You can find out more about this and other useful links for this condition at www.mind.org.uk (see also pages 78, 93 and 212).

PLANNING AHEAD
Buying bedding

If you're about to get a cot for your baby, make sure that you've got enough bedding. You'll need three cotton sheets, plus either a couple of cellular blankets (larger than the ones that fit a Moses basket) or a couple of baby sleeping bags. Don't buy duvets, quilts or pillows for your baby as he shouldn't use these until he is at least a year old. Don't use cot bumpers because your baby can get tangled up in them and even suffocate.

week 10

You will hopefully switch your baby to a cot this week because he'll be getting too big for his Moses basket, and kicking a lot more which could topple it over. If for some reason you need to use the Moses basket for a couple more weeks, put it on the floor rather than its stand as this is now too precarious. Ideally the cot should go in your bedroom because room-sharing has been shown to reduce the risk of cot death. It's best to wait until your baby is six months old before putting him in his own room.

Another milestone this week is that bathtime with your baby will start being fun – this means you can rely on his bath to distract him and to cheer him up at the end of the day when he's tired and grizzly.

You can tell from about now whether your baby's eyes are going to ultimately be brown or blue – although there are always a few surprises and the final colour isn't fully established until a baby is one, or sometimes older.

SLEEP

Total sleep required: 14–16 hours a day
Pattern: Sleeps more at night than during the day – aim for your baby to have at least five hours of uninterrupted sleep at night, plus daytime naps that total at least three hours

Your baby will look tiny when you put him in his new cot, but this doesn't mean he's too young to sleep in it. Babies can sleep in cots from birth but parents often choose a Moses basket for the convenience of being able to carry it to different rooms. Another advantage of the Moses basket is that, being small, it probably helped your baby feel secure reminding him of the confined space in the womb.

The first time you put him in his cot he'll probably cry and refuse to sleep. You will have to help him get used to his new cot by standing next to him and keeping a reassuring hand on him, perhaps gently stroking his tummy or knee. Make sure that he's relaxed and sleepy but not too fractious – perhaps try putting him in the cot after a feed.

Don't worry too much if he seems to hate his new cot, he'll get used to it after a day or two if you give plenty of reassurance and spend a little extra time settling him.

CRYING

Number of hours your baby may cry in a day:
30 minutes–3 hours

If your baby has colic, he'll still be wailing in the evenings and will continue to do so for another couple of weeks. By now you'll have perfected your soothing ritual and probably come to accept that a certain amount of crying each night is inevitable. There's one positive physiological aspect to your baby's crying, which is that stress hormones are released in tears. That's why when babies cry (and adults too for that matter) they feel less stressed and more relaxed afterwards. So while you wait for the day when your baby is over his colic, console yourself by the fact that his crying will actually be helping him through his griping pains and wind. And while on the subject of the physiological benefits of crying, it's worth noting that there is no evidence that crying is good for the lungs – as many people like to claim as they justify leaving a young baby to howl!

FEEDING

Total milk required: 720–1020 ml/24–34 oz a day
(up to 210 ml/7 oz per feed)
Pattern: 5–8 feeds a day

It's quite common around now for your baby to suddenly switch from being a hungry little feeder to a baby who really doesn't seem that bothered by food. Instead of guzzling away he'll seem distracted and keep looking about the room and be unable to concentrate on drinking his milk. This happens because his vision has developed sufficiently for him to be able to see across the room. So if there are other people around or he's somewhere different, or even if the TV is on, then he'll be far more interested in his surroundings than in feeding. To help him concentrate, you may have to take him off to the bedroom for a feed where it is quiet with no distractions.

Breastfeeding

Your baby becoming distracted is more of a problem if he is breastfed because his face is pushed up against your breast and he can't see what else is going on. He'll turn his head if he hears something interesting, which can be very painful as your nipple is suddenly yanked. To avoid this, try keeping your hand near the back of his head so that you can push him back to your breast and then un-suction him from your nipple using a finger.

As well as taking your baby to a quiet room to breastfeed, you could also try covering him with a shawl so that he can't see what's going on. This won't, however, work if you're in a noisy room because your baby will still be curious about his surroundings.

You may also find that your baby wants to suck for a minute or two, stops to look at you and perhaps smile, then returns to his meal. Although it draws out the feed, try to make the most of this stage and enjoy socialising with your baby over 'lunch'. As the novelty wears off he won't have quite so many social breaks during his meals.

Bottle-feeding

Your bottle-fed baby won't be as easily distracted as a breastfed baby because it's possible for him to feed and look around the room at the same time – you can position him sitting up on your lap with his back against you. You'll notice that for some feeds he'll want to watch his surroundings, but for others, usually at bedtime and during the night, he'll want to snuggle up against you for comfort. Like the breastfed babies, he'll probably want to 'talk' during some feeds, stopping to grin at you in between gulps of milk. Allow him to do this because mealtimes are now becoming a social event rather than just a chance to fill up.

NAPPIES

Number of wet nappies over 24 hours: 4–8
Number of dirty nappies over 24 hours: 0–5

Last week we talked about using washable nappies to help protect the environment (see page 151). But if you prefer disposables or can only cope with using washable ones for some of the time, then look out for disposable nappies that are more environmentally friendly. These will be biodegradable so will take less time decomposing in landfill sites. You can also buy biodegradable nappy bags (from Waitrose), which have the added advantage of not being scented. And never throw away plastic supermarket bags as these make good nappy bags and nappy bin liners.

Apart from making environmentally friendly nappy choices, there are plenty of other things you can do to reduce the impact your tiny baby has on the world's resources. First of all you've no doubt noticed how much extra washing you're now doing. So make sure that your washing machine is really full before you put it on as this saves energy – another energy-saving measure is not to put your machine on hotter than it needs to be. You can also use bibs to help reduce the volume of clothes to be washed.

WASHING

From this week onwards, your baby will begin to really enjoy bathtime so you could buy him some bath toys. A couple of plastic ducks will do – yellow is a primary colour, which is more interesting to your baby than pastel colours. As the ducks float, your baby will enjoy trying to bash them with his hands and feet.

DEVELOPMENT AND PLAYING

You can help your baby to build his sitting muscles by holding him under his arms and helping him to balance in the sitting position. Pull faces at him to encourage your baby to lift his head, but don't play the sitting game for longer than a couple of minutes because he'll become tired.

This week you can be fairly sure whether your baby will have blue or brown eyes, although you won't yet know the final shade as they will continue to darken until your baby is one, or sometimes older. So if your baby has brown or brown-green eyes they will almost certainly stay dark. And if your baby's eyes are blue then they are likely to end up blue, blue-green or grey.

Up until now, your baby has not been able to see in three dimensions and has had a rather flat view of the world. This is because he has viewed two slightly different images from each eye, so his brain has had to suppress one of these images to stop him seeing double. But now your baby's brain is able to mesh the two images together, which means that three-dimensional vision is fully developed. This will enable your baby to bash at his toys more precisely.

!SAFETY TIP OF THE WEEK!
Don't leave your baby alone in the car

If your baby is asleep in the back of the car it can be extremely tempting to leave him while you whiz into a shop rather than disturb him and have to fuss about transferring him into his pram. But you should never leave your baby alone in the car because of the risk of abduction, and also the more likely risk of heatstroke. Cars can become extremely hot in the summer, even with the windows open.

WHEN TO SEE A DOCTOR

Meningitis

Meningitis is when the lining of the brain becomes infected. Although this disease is extremely serious it is also extremely rare. Your baby has now had his first round in immunisation against *Haemophilus influenzae* Type B (Hib), plus the pneumococcal jab which gives him some protection against meningitis. He will soon have his first meningitis C vaccine, but this won't protect him against all types of meningitis or septicaemia (blood poisoning which can be caused by the meningitis bacteria), so it's important to know the symptoms because your baby can become very ill within a few hours.

Symptoms include refusing to feed, a fever, irritability and vomiting, all of which can occur when your baby has a cold which can make meningitis difficult to spot. But your baby may also seem listless, be very pale and have mottled skin, have cold hands, and foot or leg pain. These symptoms can develop after just eight hours of the illness striking. Then after about 12 to 24 hours, you may notice your baby becoming sensitive to light, and having a high-pitched cry that gets worse when you pick him up because he has a headache. He may also develop a rash anywhere on his body – see the 'glass test' opposite.

If your baby has just one or two of these symptoms and you instinctively know that he is ill, then take him along to the hospital Emergency Department, where the doctors will be only too happy to check him out, and with luck give him the all-clear. The worst thing you can do is to delay getting medical help because meningitis can become lethal within hours – don't take any chances by waiting around for more conclusive symptoms as this could potentially cost your child's life. And if you are sent home but your baby becomes worse, don't feel embarrassed about taking him back again for another check.

If doctors suspect meningitis, they will do a lumbar puncture (put a small needle into his back to tap the fluid around his brain) and your baby will be given intravenous antibiotics (via a drip put into the back of his hand) as a precaution while the doctors wait for test results. Bacterial meningitis requires a prolonged course of antibiotics and it can take a couple of months for your baby to recover. He will be given a hearing test to rule out deafness, the most treatable complication. And other complications, including cerebral palsy (some degree of paralysis) and moderate learning difficulties, will hopefully be ruled out as your baby gets older.

The Meningitis Research Foundation has a free 24-hour helpline (080 8800 3344) or visit www.meningitis.org.

The glass test

The meningococcal infection can cause blood poisoning – septicaemia – which shows up as red or purple spots. These do not fade under pressure so you can put a clear drinking glass over the rash and press it against your baby's skin to see if the rash becomes less red. If it doesn't fade then take your baby to your hospital's Emergency Department immediately. But please note that children can be extremely ill with meningitis and yet have no rash whatsoever – so don't wait around for a rash to appear before seeking medical help.

WHAT'S HAPPENING TO MUM

By now, your abdominal muscles will have begun to fuse together again and be much stronger – this is the first step to regaining a flat stomach. You can strengthen them further by doing some sit-ups, but don't attempt these if the gap between the muscles is still bigger than two fingers wide. To measure your gap, lie on your back with your knees bent and lift your head. You'll feel your abdominal muscles coming together as you lift and it should feel almost closed before you do any sit-ups.

PLANNING AHEAD
Immunisations

Make sure that your baby is booked in for his second lot of jabs, due at three months of age (see page 133). This is for meningitis C plus the five-in-one DtaP/IPV/Hib vaccine and is the second part of the immunisation course, which began a couple of weeks ago. If your baby's first immunisations were delayed because he had a fever, then make sure there is a four-week gap until his second round.

week 11

This week, even the most difficult babies will be sleeping more deeply, crying less, and having a fairly regular feeding pattern. Some babies fall into this more mature pattern when they're just a few weeks old, most start to adopt it by eight weeks, and the late developers take until now.

Whatever your baby has been like in the early weeks, you can look forward to easier times ahead – colic is about to disappear, which marks the end of evening crying, and babies are less sensitive to every little change that can upset them in the early days. Your baby will also seem more robust to handle now that he's bigger and will have lost that spindly newborn physique – this of course makes dressing and bathing him easier.

SLEEP

Total sleep required: 14–16 hours a day
Pattern: sleeps more at night than during the day – aim for your baby to have at least five hours of uninterrupted sleep at night, plus daytime naps that total at least three hours

HOW TO REDUCE NIGHT-TIME AWAKENINGS

1. Keep the bedroom dark because your baby may well open his eyes for a few seconds during his lighter sleep phase.
2. Don't rush to pick him up the moment he stirs because this is guaranteed to waken him fully – it's normal for babies to moan and cry a little, and even to open their eyes, and yet still remain asleep. So allow a few minutes to make a decision about whether or not to feed or cuddle your baby because there's still a chance that he will drop back off again by himself.
3. Keep the noise down – most noises will wake a sensitive baby during his light sleep, other babies may be able to sleep through familiar noises but will be startled by something more unusual like an alarm. Once your baby is breathing softly and not moving, he's in his deep sleep cycle so you can make quite a lot of noise without waking him. But if he's shuffling around his cot he's probably in his lighter sleep phase so take care not to wake him. Some parents make a point of not tiptoeing around when their baby is asleep in order to get him used to sleeping through noise. If you do this then you are bound to wake him up a few times before he becomes used to noise, but it's worth the effort because he will become less noise-sensitive.

By now, your baby's sleep cycle has lengthened from 40 minutes when he was first born to an hour. This means that he now only rouses into light sleep every hour and spends the rest of the cycle in a deep, dreamless sleep during which virtually nothing will wake him. Eventually your baby's sleep cycle will be 90 minutes, like an adult's, but for now, he spends a lot more of the night in a light sleep than you, which is why he is so easily disturbed.

Some anthropologists have theorised that sleeping lightly is a protection mechanism to ensure that babies don't die from starvation or exposure during the night – they're programmed to wake frequently and cry if they need anything. That's all very well, but babies also wake up for no reason at all, which is why it's important to teach your baby to stop waking up fully during his light sleep phases. Eventually he won't even wake up to be fed and then, like an adult, he'll have a few moments each night when he wakes briefly and goes straight back to sleep – he won't even remember waking by the morning.

CRYING

Number of hours your baby may cry in a day:
30 minutes–3 hours

Weaning your baby off his dummy

If your baby has a dummy, ideally try to wean him off it around now before he becomes too set in his ways. It's more difficult to break habits once your baby is three months old so if you can bear it, tackle the dummy addiction now. The first time you gave your baby a dummy, probably when he was about a month old, you no doubt had good intentions about only using it for a few weeks and limiting its use to when your baby cried hard and needed to calm down for a sleep. You may even have intended to remove it just before he fell asleep to avoid it becoming a sleep prop that would have to be taken away at a later stage. If you've managed to stick to these restrictions, your baby is probably not using his dummy often anyway, and when you take it away completely it shouldn't cause him too much distress. But it's more likely that your baby now needs his dummy for sleeping and that the thought of weaning him off it fills you with dread as you wonder how on earth you'll get him to stop crying and sleep without it.

Well, the good news is that research suggests that dummies reduce the risk of cot death as they stop babies sleeping so deeply. And the scientists even suggest that 'forgetting' to give your baby his dummy ups his risk of cot death more than if he had never used a dummy in the first place. So you have the perfect excuse to delay the dummy ban. But in the meantime, you could try limiting your baby's dummy for sleeping only, and not take it with you when you go out. Yes, he'll howl in supermarkets and you'll have to be more organised about feeding him because you won't be able to buy five minutes' grace with the dummy, but he will soon learn to sleep in his pram without the dummy. This shouldn't take more than about a week as he's still very young, and also the movement of the pram compensates for the lack of dummy.

When you do decide to stop the dummy altogether, the quickest way is to go cold turkey. Your baby will be distraught for up to a week, with the first three nights being particularly tough. Alternatively you can reduce the use of the dummy gradually, perhaps taking it out of your baby's mouth once he's asleep, and taking it away during the day. A good time to stop the dummy altogether is somewhere between six months (from then on the risk of cot death is minimal) and a year (after this your baby will become increasingly wilful). Don't delay it until after the age of two or you really will have a battle on your hands.

FEEDING

Total milk required: 720–1080 ml/24–36 oz a day
(up to 210 ml/7 oz per feed)
Pattern: 5–8 feeds a day

Whether bottle- or breastfeeding, you won't be feeling anxious any more about whether you're doing it right, or if your baby is having enough milk. So now is a good time to think about getting organised and making your life more convenient. If you are breastfeeding, think about freezing your milk, or if you are bottle-feeding, packing up powdered milk portions for when you are out. Both of these are fiddly, which is why it probably wasn't worth worrying about before now.

Breastfeeding

You might want to build up a milk bank if you are going back to work and don't want your baby to drink any formula. The best time to express is in the morning as this is when you have the most milk, and try to express after a feed so that your baby doesn't go short. You can pump as often as you like, but remember that you will increase your milk supply after a few days so you will no longer have the finely tuned balance of supply and demand with your baby. For this reason it makes sense to build up your milk stock slowly, which is possible as frozen milk keeps for a couple of months.

You'll need a breast pump (see page 25), and also ice-cube trays for freezing. You can pour your milk into sterilised ice-cube trays, about an ounce per tray, then transfer the frozen cubes into plastic bags. To thaw the cubes, put the required number into a sterilised bottle then place this in a bowl of hot water to defrost. Don't re-freeze the milk once it has thawed. If you express milk while you are away from the home, you'll need to refrigerate it and carry it home in a cool pack. If you decide that expressing is not worth the bother, then don't feel guilty because breast milk actually loses a lot of its nutritional value once it has been frozen. So there's little difference between formula and frozen breast milk.

Bottle-feeding

When you're out with your baby, you have a number of feeding options. You can make up bottles at home and keep these in a cool pack – the disadvantage is that this is heavy to carry. Another option is to use cartons of ready-made formula – this is the most expensive option and again heavy to carry. Or you could use powdered milk – this comes in sachets for travelling, which saves you having to keep it in a special container. Sachets, however, are a more expensive way of buying powdered milk than a tin.

The cheapest choice is to use powdered milk from a large tin – measure out the exact amount your baby needs for a feed before you set off and put the powder into a plastic, lidded container. You can buy specially designed containers that have three compartments for up to three feeds, and a small lid that makes pouring the powder into a bottle easy. Then you just add pre-boiled water when you are out. This requires a bit of initial organisation but is the most economical option. (Avent make these containers and they are available from large pharmacies.)

Hopefully your baby doesn't need his milk to be warmed up any more, but if he is fussy about the temperature, you'll need to heat up his formula when you're out and about. Ask in restaurants and cafés for a bowl of hot water and, as always, test the milk before giving it to your baby. The other option is to take a flask of hot water, pour it into the bottle and allow it to cool to the correct temperature before adding the powder.

Finally, remember to keep teats sterile by using protective caps, and keep sterilised bottles and teats in plastic bags in your baby bag in a separate compartment to the nappies and changing mat.

NAPPIES

Number of wet nappies over 24 hours: 4–8
Number of dirty nappies over 24 hours: 0–5

Nappies won't seem to dominate your life any more because you'll be quick at changing a nappy, and also you'll no longer be changing nappies at night as your baby is unlikely to be pooing at that time. There will, of course, be the odd exception.

Not only will your baby be having fewer bowel movements, but when he does go to the toilet he won't be straining excessively because his anus muscles are pretty much fully developed. If he does start straining and finds going to the toilet painful, it probably means that he's constipated (see page 116).

Another change that makes nappies less of an issue these days is that your baby will rarely wee while you're changing him, so you don't often have to go through the bother of cleaning him up and changing all his clothes. He isn't weeing as frequently as he used to because his bladder is getting bigger in size and holding more urine.

WASHING

Assuming that your baby now enjoys his bath, you might want to think about building his confidence in water. The key is not to be overcautious and to enjoy lots of splashing – this is where dad comes into his own. It's really not a problem if your baby gets water over his face and in his eyes – it won't do him any harm and if you are relaxed and laughing he'll be happy enough. If your baby doesn't yet love bathtime, then wait a few weeks before being too boisterous with him.

DEVELOPMENT AND PLAYING

Your baby will continue to practise reaching for his baby gym or toys strung across his cot or pram, and you'll see him getting better at hitting his targets by the day. He still can't reach for an object in one clean movement, because the messaging system between his brain, eyes and arm is still developing so he will use lots of jerky movements.

By now your baby's neck muscles are quite strong so that, when you hold him, he can hold his head up easily and look around the room. And when he's on his front, he may be able to push his chest off the floor while he has a quick look around, before collapsing again.

! SAFETY TIP OF THE WEEK !
Painkillers

Never give your baby adult painkillers such as paracetamol. If you run out of Calpol and your baby has a temperature or is feeling unwell after his immunisations, you may be tempted to try to give him a tiny dose of an adult paracetamol tablet. DON'T – this is extremely dangerous because an adult tablet contains nearly 10 times the amount of paracetamol that is safe to give your baby. So it would be impossible to cut the tablet up accurately and small enough. And never give him adult liquid medicines either – wait until you can get to a chemist and buy the special baby medicines.

WHEN TO SEE A DOCTOR

Coughing

When your baby gets a cough it's natural to feel a bit anxious and to worry that there's something seriously wrong. But the most common reason for a cough is the common cold (see page 43) which can irritate the airways if there's a lot of mucus. Such coughs are generally self-limiting and nothing to worry about even though they're chesty and sometimes persist for more than a week. Assuming your baby is feeding well, seems happy and doesn't have a fever, there's no need to see your doctor. But if your baby's cough becomes worse, starts keeping him awake at night, and he develops a fever and goes off his food, then see your GP. Your baby may have a chest infection which can be treated with antibiotics.

Pneumonia

Rarely, a chesty cough develops into pneumonia, which is very serious. The most distinctive symptom is rapid breathing (nearly one breath per second), listlessness and poor feeding. Your baby will also have an alarming sounding chesty cough, a fever, chest pain, poor feeding and be listless. Very occasionally a baby with pneumonia will cough up blood.

Whooping cough

This is rare as most babies are now vaccinated against whooping cough (see page 133). But the illness begins like the common cold, followed by violent coughing fits during which he will fight desperately for breath. Get immediate medical help because whooping cough can be fatal. These attacks can occur in the first couple of weeks, then the child is left with a persistent cough that lasts for up to three months.

Croup

This is a viral infection that attacks the vocal cords resulting in a rasping seal-like barking cough and a noisy in-breath. Despite this frightening cough, it's essential that you don't panic so that you can keep your baby calm – if he's relaxed then his airways will relax and open more. You can also take him into the bathroom and run a bath to create a steamy environment which will give him some relief.

A bit of rasping at night if your baby is able to sleep isn't a medical emergency. But if you think that your baby is finding it difficult to breathe then get immediate medical help.

Bronchiolitis

This common viral infection (see page 210) causes a wet, chesty cough that can last for several weeks. Generally it's nothing to worry about unless your baby seems very unwell with a fever and feeding difficulties, in which case see your doctor.

HOMEOPATHY

There are lots of homeopathic remedies to treat different types of cough. By all means try these but don't rely on them to the extent that you delay taking your child to see a doctor. If your baby has a chesty cough with a fever, or shows any signs of breathing difficulties, then see your GP right away because bacterial infections left untreated can sometimes become life-threatening. You may well be worried about your child being put on antibiotics, but your doctor will only prescribe these if absolutely necessary.

WHAT'S HAPPENING TO MUM

By now, your body will be pretty much back to normal and you can start strenuous exercise. Start slowly and build up as it can take up to five months for your ligaments to completely return to their pre-birth state. Remember that even if you used to be fit you will find that it takes about another three months before you are training at full strength. Be particularly careful with high-impact exercises – those where you take both feet off the ground, such as running, skipping and aerobics. Some women prefer to wait until five months after giving birth to do such exercises.

PLANNING AHEAD
Shop for milk storage containers

Spend some time shopping for the right equipment for either freezing expressed milk, or transporting formula when you're out and about. Your baby will drink either breast or formula milk until he's one so it's worth forking out now for the right gear because it will save you money in the long term. It will mean that either you won't have to buy formula milk at all, or that you won't have to pay a premium for convenience products such as cartons of milk.

week 12

Three months marks the unofficial rite of passage when your baby is no longer a helpless little creature. Instead of craving a recreation of his womb environment, he embraces the outside world and becomes a bouncing, gurgling flirt whose sole purpose appears to be to befriend everyone he sees.

Up until this point you will have done your best to attend to your baby's every need, but now you can relax a little because he'll be a lot less demanding – wanting fewer feeds and nappy changes, as well as sleeping more easily at night. So this is a very good time to start thinking about sleep training if you've not done so already. It's still easy to establish new habits with your baby but from now on he'll become gradually more set in his ways, which means that it's important to get him into good, rather than bad, habits.

Your baby is also likely to go through his third growth spurt around now so prepare for him to be ravenous. And this week is also when he's due for his second lot of immunisations, assuming he began his first batch at eight weeks.

SLEEP

Total sleep required: 14–16 hours a day
Pattern: aim for your baby to have at least five hours of uninterrupted sleep at night, plus daytime naps that total at least three hours

From around the time your baby is three months old, you can start to look forward to getting a bit more sleep. It's still far too soon to be putting your baby to bed and forgetting about him until morning, but 70 per cent of babies of this age will sleep for five hours or more at some stage during the night.

If your baby is having five hours of uninterrupted sleep at night then, medically speaking, he is sleeping 'through the night'. Of course, a doctor's definition of 'through the night' differs from a parent's, and you are no doubt expecting that your baby will eventually sleep for about 12 hours at night. This will happen, but not yet. If your baby isn't having a five-hour chunk of night-sleep, it could be that he doesn't weigh enough to be able to go this long without food – babies should weigh at least 5 kg/11 lb to go for five hours and not eat.

Assuming that your baby is heavy enough, then you can gently steer him towards having a lengthy night's sleep by making sure he's having enough feeds during the day, and also ensuring that he's not in the habit of needing milk to settle himself when he surfaces from light sleep. If this is the case you need to stop your baby falling asleep during feeds (see page 136).

Don't be too disheartened if your baby isn't yet able to sleep for five hours during the night as most babies sort themselves out eventually, and up to 80 per cent of all nine-month-old babies can sleep for at least five hours at night.

CRYING

Number of hours your baby may cry in a day: 1 hour

If your baby has suffered from colic, you will soon be celebrating because your baby's endless crying sessions will come to an abrupt end either this week or next. Most babies don't cry nearly as much once they reach three months, and when your baby does cry, you'll probably find it easier to work out why.

Even if your baby hasn't suffered from colic, you'll still appreciate an improvement as your baby will cry considerably less than in the early weeks – some babies cry for as little as five minutes a day, although about an hour in total is average.

There are a few exceptions and some babies will continue to cry a lot for no particular reason. If you're concerned then seek advice. If nothing else this will give you peace of mind.

FEEDING

Total milk required: 720–1200 ml/24–40 oz a day
(up to 210 ml/7 oz per feed)
Pattern: 5–8 feeds a day

Most babies have a growth spurt at around three months, so be prepared for your baby not only to be hungry but also to be more tired and fractious than usual. As with previous growth spurts, this will be hard work if you are breastfeeding because your milk supply will need to increase. So be prepared to put your feet up for a couple of days and allow your baby to feed as often as he likes. This may feel as though you're returning to the haphazard early days of having absolutely no structure or routine to your day, but go with it because it is only temporary while your milk production increases.

If you are bottle-feeding, follow your baby's lead and increase his milk accordingly – it's likely that he'll want an extra couple of ounces or so a day, perhaps more. After this growth spurt, milk intake tends to plateau and will increase more steadily than it has done over the first three months.

WASHING

Last week we talked about building your baby's confidence in water during bathtime. To continue this theme you might want to try sloshing a handful of water over his head and face. When you do this, say his name, and then say 'weee' as you scoop the water over him. He'll recognise this as a cue and eventually learn to shut his eyes and mouth. As well as teaching your baby to enjoy water, this will also make future hair-washing sessions easy – these can become extremely difficult because most toddlers hate having water in their eyes unless they have become used to it.

If your baby does happen to take in a mouthful of bath water and end up coughing and spluttering, stay calm, hold him steady while he clears his airways, and if he seems upset or frightened then whiz him out of the bath and cuddle him close in a towel while he recovers. The important thing is that you don't panic – it's not dangerous for your baby to splutter on bath water.

DEVELOPMENT AND PLAYING

Your baby may start to rock when he's lying on his back by bringing his knees up to his chest and swinging from side to side. This is to prepare him to roll over in a couple of months and, in the meantime, allows him to shuffle around in circles and see the room from different angles. Put him on a soft rug with plenty of space around him.

Your baby may chuckle for the first time this week and you can encourage his giggles by gently tickling him, blowing raspberries, and doing pretend sneezes and comedy coughing. Of course if you laugh and smile a lot yourself, you'll encourage him to join in.

WHEN TO SEE A DOCTOR

Wheezing

It can be very alarming to hear your baby making a strange wheezing
noise every time he breathes out, but wheezing is actually quite
common from between weeks 12 and 20. Your first concern may be
that your baby has developed asthma. The good news is that wheezing
in babies usually disappears as your baby gets older and his lungs
mature. Having said that, wheezing can mean that asthma will be
diagnosed, usually at around two years, but most wheezing babies
won't go on to develop this condition.

Up to a quarter of all children under five will develop a viral-
induced wheeze – this is three times more common in boys – and
wheezing can last for a couple of months. Passive smoking can make
babies more susceptible to developing a viral wheeze because their
lungs may have reduced capacity. Bronchiolitis (see page 210) can
also cause a persistent wheeze that can go on for weeks.

Allergies are unlikely to be the cause of wheezing at this age because babies rarely develop a reaction to cats, grass, dust or other environmental triggers before they are at least nine months old. If your child's wheezing is triggered by an allergy, he may take longer to grow out of it.

Treatment

Get any wheezing checked by your doctor, who may prescribe Atrovent and/or Ventolin, which are used to treat asthma and other breathing problems. You can give these to your baby using an asthma inhaler together with something called a spacer device – this is a large plastic container attached to a face mask which fits over your baby's nose and mouth (see below).

As well as giving your baby medicine to help his wheezing, there are measures you can take yourself, including breastfeeding your baby which has been shown to reduce his risk of asthma. Avoiding smoky atmospheres also helps, as does giving up smoking.

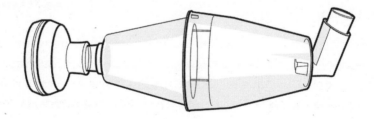

A spacer device fits over your baby's nose and mouth so that he can inhale medicine to ease wheezing.

WHAT'S HAPPENING TO MUM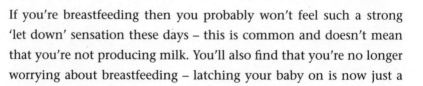

If you're breastfeeding then you probably won't feel such a strong 'let down' sensation these days – this is common and doesn't mean that you're not producing milk. You'll also find that you're no longer worrying about breastfeeding – latching your baby on is now just a matter of sticking his head under your t-shirt and letting him get on with it.

You've also got plenty of milk, which means that expressing is unlikely to upset the delicate balance between supply and demand too much. So it's probably time to get pumping and go out for an evening – if you haven't done so already of course. Keep your phone on but do try to resist calling every half hour because, although hard to imagine, your baby really will be perfectly okay without you.

Make sure you go out with your partner. Even though you'll probably talk to each other about your baby and not much else for most of the night, being alone together will help you recall some of those distant memories of when you were a 'normal' couple and didn't squabble over who's more tired and whose turn it is to get up for the baby.

PLANNING AHEAD
Buying a travel cot

If you're thinking about buying a travel cot, now is a good time because your baby is quite portable and easy to travel with at the moment. He's old enough not to be waking every couple of hours at night and yet still young enough not to notice too much that he's sleeping somewhere else.

The sooner you buy your cot, the more use you will get out of it. You can justify the expense because the cot will double up as a playpen, which will be invaluable in a few months' time when your baby is mobile and you need to leave him somewhere safe while, say, you rush to the loo. When buying a travel cot look for one that is light and compact enough for you to carry when folded, but also sturdy enough for a boisterous toddler when erected. It's also important that you're able to set it up properly, as some people find certain models fiddly. Try a dry run in the shop before you buy.

week 13

Over the last three months there have probably been times when you've spent almost the entire day with your baby in your arms because he seemed particularly fretful. Or you may have tucked him into your bed when you felt desperate and unable to face the long drawn-out process of trying to settle him back into his cot. Some people would say that you've 'spoilt' your baby and that he would have fared better with a timetabled no-nonsense regime. They may even suggest that your baby is crafty and has you wrapped around his little finger. Ignore them. Babies aren't manipulative – far from it. They simply cry when they want something because this is their only means of communication. If you've cosseted your baby over the past weeks, then congratulations because most experts are now convinced that lots of cuddling will help your baby to grow up to be secure.

Although you should continue to 'spoil' your baby, it's important not to allow him to slip into unacceptable habits such as feeding every two hours throughout the night. The next few months are critical for helping your baby to develop good sleeping and feeding habits. His body will naturally demand more sleep at night and if you can avoid allowing him to get into bad habits you should be on the home straight for teaching him to sleep through the night.

SLEEP

Total sleep required: 14–16 hours a day
Pattern: aim for your baby to have at least five hours of uninterrupted sleep at night, daytime naps that total at least three hours, and for him to go to bed early

From this week you can reclaim your evenings as you start putting your baby to bed nice and early. This is now possible because he will no longer be crying from colic or general evening fussiness, and he will also become sleepy in the evenings and stop getting that curious burst of night energy that can make new babies suddenly sociable at about 9pm. We suggested in week four that you introduced a bedtime routine (see page 81), but now you will find that your baby is much more willing to go to sleep earlier. What you're aiming for is to have a routine of say a bath, nappy, song, feed, cuddle and a kiss goodnight. Then to be able to put your baby in his cot, walk out of the room and for him to fall asleep about 10 minutes later.

Choose a bedtime when your baby naturally seems to get sleepy for the night then follow the routine at the same time each evening. You'll notice that after about four days your baby will recognise his bedtime cues and know that it's time to go to sleep, so by the time you put him in his cot he's already feeling sleepy. You can then bring bedtime forward by about 20 minutes and do so every few days until you've reached your chosen bedtime. Some parents aim for 7pm, others prefer 8pm so that they can spend time with their baby when they get home from work. Whatever time you decide, it's easy enough to change at a later date – after all when the clocks go back parents manage to adjust their babies' body clocks pretty swiftly.

If your baby doesn't settle or wakes up too soon

Reading the theory is one thing, but putting the bedtime regime into practice takes patience, perseverance and time. Bedtime is one of the most challenging aspects of your child's sleep training and putting the effort in now will pay dividends in the future when your toddler settles down to bed without a fuss.

When you begin bedtime training, your baby is unlikely to go off to sleep when you put him in his cot. And when he does finally settle, he will almost certainly wake up again about an hour later. The first thing to do is wait five minutes to ensure that your baby isn't having a pre-sleep moan – don't leave him to cry hard for more than a few minutes because he's too young for full blown sleep training and controlled crying. When you're sure that he's not going to drift off to sleep by himself, try to soothe him to sleep by doing as little as possible – so choose 'minimum soothers' from the box below in preference to the 'maximum soothers'. You may find that during the first week of early nights, your baby is difficult to soothe and that you have to resort to the maximum soothers. Don't worry, the important thing is to teach his body to feel tired in the evenings. Once you've got your baby's physiology sorted out it will be easier to work on his psychology because he'll feel genuinely tired and respond better as you reduce the amount of help you give him getting to sleep.

Next week we cover reasons that your baby may not be settling to sleep in the evenings, but in the meantime, see the box below for a step by step guide to soothing your baby to sleep.

SOOTHING YOUR BABY TO SLEEP

Aim to gradually use more of the minimum soothers rather than the maximum ones. And eventually don't use anything at all – just let your baby drop off by himself.

Maximum soothers
• Turning a side lamp on

- Feeding him
- Singing to him
- Rocking him
- Cheering him up so that he stops crying
- Putting him in your bed
- Cuddling him until he drops off to sleep

Minimum soothers
- Keeping the light off
- Quiet sshing sounds
- Stroking him while he's in his cot
- Standing or sitting next to the cot not touching him, but allowing him to see that you are there

FEEDING

Total milk required: 720–1200 ml/24–40 oz a day (up to 210 ml/7 oz per feed)
Pattern: 5–8 feeds a day

If you're breastfeeding, you may notice around now that your baby begins to be less interested in feeding during the day but seems increasingly hungry at night. This happens for a number of reasons – perhaps you're very busy in the day, particularly if you have other children. The result could be that you don't spend as much time feeding your baby as he would like, his feeds get interrupted by siblings wanting your attention, and his milk times may even get a bit delayed if you're very busy. But at night your baby has you all to himself and can have long, undisturbed feeds with mum.

Another reason for daytime feeding to decline is that your baby is distracted by what's going on around him and is less interested in snuggling down for long feeds than he used to be. Again, night-time is when he catches up by drinking extra milk when there are no distractions.

Also if you're out and about more these days this can delay feeds, and if you are feeding in cafés or when you're with friends, you may feel a bit self-conscious and cut the feed short. If you recognise this pattern developing then try to stop it now because if you let it go on, you'll find that your baby's appetite decreases drastically during the day and he's ravenous for most of the night.

Reversing the night-time ravenous pattern

The easiest way to change the pattern is to ensure that you are feeding your baby enough during the day, then he should stop being quite so hungry at night. So watch the clock, feed him regularly and also take the time to have quiet private feeds with no distractions. If this doesn't seem to have much effect then you will have to cut back on your baby's night feeds to no more than once every four hours in order to increase his daytime hunger. It may take a few nights for this new feeding regime to have an impact on your baby's daytime appetite and it will be tough as he screams for food while you watch the clock and wait for the hours to pass (you or your partner can cuddle him while you wait). But this will get results and reverse his day–night feeding patterns. This problem may occur again when you start your baby on solids (see page 214).

NAPPIES

Number of wet nappies over 24 hours: 4–8
Number of dirty nappies over 24 hours: 0–5

By now you will be able to change nappies with lightning speed and with minimal fuss and mess. But being on nappy autopilot will increase the likelihood that you forget to wash your hands after a nappy change. It's essential that you never forget, because a tiny bit of poo on your fingers can easily transfer a bug to your baby via his mouth and give him diarrhoea.

If you notice other people forgetting to wash their hands, perhaps your partner, the babysitter or granny – just go ahead and remind them. They might fume with indignation, but this is preferable to your baby becoming ill.

From this week we won't be covering nappies as a separate section because very little changes. The exception is when your baby starts on solids, so we've included a final nappy section in week 17.

WASHING

If your baby has become used to you splashing water gently over his face at bathtime, then you could step things up a bit and start using a small cup as this will further encourage water confidence. Do this every day and remember to warn your baby by saying his name then saying 'weee', or whatever you decide is an appropriate warning that you are about to tip water over his head. The important thing is to be consistent, make it fun and keep bathtime nice and boisterous. It's essential that your baby continues to enjoy his bathtime and that you don't push him too hard with these water games. If he's surprised that's fine, but make sure that he doesn't become frightened.

DEVELOPMENT AND PLAYING

By now your baby has completely lost his grasp reflex, which means that he holds his hands open instead of in fists. If you put your finger in his palm he'll clutch it because he's chosen to, not because it's a reflex response. He'll also let go when he wants to – previously you had to prise things away from his fists, or wait until his hands became tired.

If you use a baby carrier, you can turn your baby to face outwards as he now has enough head control to be comfortable in this new position. He's also very curious about the outside world and will love seeing it from an upright position. When it's time for his nap, it's easy enough to turn him back round again to face you.

Your baby is old enough to like some people more than others and shows his preference with his smiles. He will smile broadly at people he recognises and loves, and reserve a smaller smile for those he doesn't know. As he gets used to new people, he'll soon start beaming.

!SAFETY TIP OF THE WEEK!
Don't attend to your baby while driving

When you're in the car, resist the temptation to turn around and help your baby if he starts crying. Even if he's howling at full throttle, there's little you can do while you're driving apart from talk to him. Remind yourself that he's perfectly safe in his car seat and try to stay focused on the road until you can find somewhere to pull over.

WHEN TO SEE A DOCTOR

Cross-eyed

Many babies appear to be cross-eyed in the first three months because their eyes don't yet move together. But from around now, your baby shouldn't look as though he has a squint because his eye muscles should be developed enough to work together. If he remains cross-eyed, it may be because he is short-sighted and unable to focus properly, in which case he needs glasses to help the eyes to realign. Even babies who are just a few months old can have glasses. It's important that your baby's squint is treated because his depth of vision may not develop properly otherwise. He may also have to do eye exercises to strengthen the muscles – these will probably involve covering one eye while showing him objects to look at with the other eye.

WHAT'S HAPPENING TO MUM

You've probably found a post-natal group by now and have met some other mums. But to extend your social circle and get your shape back at the same time, you could join a buggy fitness group. Popping up around the country are groups of women pacing round parks with their prams and buggies, interspersed with sessions of lunges and squats.

These classes have even been shown to beat the blues – research published in the *International Journal of Nursing Practice* found that women diagnosed with post natal depression (see page 93) had fewer symptoms if they did a 12-week buggy class than if they joined a mum and baby coffee group. See www.buggyfit.co.uk for your nearest class, or ask at your local gym or leisure centre.

PLANNING AHEAD
Book your baby's vaccinations

Make sure that your baby is booked in for his third lot of jabs, due at four months of age (see page 133). This is for meningitis C plus the five-in-one vaccine. After this, your baby has no more vaccinations until he is a year old.

week 14

Now that your baby has grown out of the colic and evening fussing stage, you'll have more time and energy to focus on his sleeping habits as you yearn for an uninterrupted night's sleep. This week we continue with the bedtime theme because this is such an important part of your baby's sleep schedule – basically if you can sort out bedtime, the rest of your baby's sleep pattern falls into place a lot more easily.

Even if you've decided to take a more relaxed approach to your baby's sleep patterns and you don't want to push him into a sleeping routine, you will find that he's becoming naturally more tired in the evenings from around this week, and that he seems to sleep more deeply at night. It's still too soon for your baby to be sleeping through the night, but the majority of parents will certainly be getting a much better night's rest than when their baby was just a couple of weeks old.

SLEEP

Total sleep required: 14–16 hours a day
*Pattern: aim for your baby to have at least five hours of
uninterrupted sleep at night, daytime naps that total at least
three hours, and for him to go to bed early*

Last week we talked about establishing a fixed bedtime (see page 185).
If you haven't yet made much progress then take heart because it
can take weeks and sometimes months before your baby consistently
settles at bedtime. But it's worth persevering because bedtime is the
foundation of your child's sleep pattern and if you can get him into
good habits at this age, things will certainly be a lot easier when he's
older. In the meantime, here are some of the things that could cause
bedtime problems.

Napping too late

Ensure that your baby wakes from his final nap at least two hours
before bedtime, otherwise he might simply feel too wide awake to
want to go to sleep. Eventually there should be a three-hour gap
between waking from his final nap and going to bed.

Adrenaline burst

Keep the hour before you put your baby to bed as calm as possible
and try to stop your baby from becoming either extremely angry or
excited. The idea is to prevent him from producing a burst of adren-
aline because this hormone will energise your baby and stop him
sleeping for at least an hour.

Dirty nappy

If your baby does a poo, it could make him uncomfortable and stop
him going off to sleep. You'll find that the older he gets the more

aware he becomes of having a dirty nappy so this is always something to check if he's not dropping off. Evening poos tend to be quite unusual, so if your baby needs his nappy changed late in the evening it will hopefully be a one-off reason for him not settling.

Overtired

If you put your baby to bed late for some reason, perhaps you've been out, then you'll find that it can take him longer to go to sleep. This happens partly because he misses his sleep window when he feels tired as the lights go off, and also because he's become overtired and so feels anxious and wound up instead of calm and sleepy. All you can do is to follow his bedtime routine as usual but perhaps speed it up a little. Then be prepared to give him some extra help getting to sleep, say stroking his back and spending a bit of time soothing him.

FEEDING

*Total milk required: 720–1200 ml/24–40 oz a day
(up to 210 ml/7 oz per feed)*
Pattern: 5–8 feeds a day

By now your baby is probably having between one and three feeds a night, one of which may be at around midnight. One question you've probably asked yourself is whether to wake your baby for a feed when you go to bed. In many ways this seems like a sensible option because filling your baby up with milk will hopefully ensure that he goes for a good few hours before needing another feed, allowing you more sleep. He may even wake one less time during the night. If this works for you then good – continue to encourage your baby to have a feed when you go to bed. But there are a number of reasons why it might not work. Firstly, your baby may wake up fully then take ages to settle. Or he might not want to wake at all and you won't manage to feed him. You might even find that waking your baby for a bedtime feed makes the rest of the night more disturbed rather than less. This can happen because by waking him, you've disturbed his basic circadian rhythm. So if his sleep–wake cycle is out of sync, it could upset his entire night's sleep. There's also the problem of a full stomach causing indigestion and a full bladder causing a leaky nappy – both of these will of course upset your baby's sleep.

If you find that this late night feed doesn't seem to help your baby to have a peaceful night then don't persevere – you'll have to drop this feed at a later stage anyway and there's no point in creating a learned expectation for an extra night feed in the meantime.

WASHING

Assuming that your baby is still happy enough during bathtime and coping well with having a small cup of water tipped over his head, you can try a bigger cup of water – aim for the size of a large yoghurt pot. An added benefit of all this bathtime splashing is that being confident in water will help your baby learn to swim. Babies and toddlers can't swim with their heads above water because their heads are too big in proportion to their bodies, so they can only swim underwater. These bathtime sessions will put your baby at a huge advantage should you decide to take him to baby swimming lessons later on (see page 198).

DEVELOPMENT AND PLAYING

Your baby is likely to start making strange high-pitched squawks this week – sounding a bit like a dinosaur – and you'll notice that he's really starting to enjoy his own voice as he experiments with different sounds.

Daily practice at reaching out for toys over the last few weeks has paid off and your baby's movements are now much smoother than they were. He'll start to actually grasp the toys any day now.

When you hold your baby in the 'standing' position, you'll notice that his legs are now strong enough to support his weight. Instead of crumpling, his legs now stiffen and straighten to take his body weight as he prepares to eventually stand and walk.

!SAFETY TIP OF THE WEEK!
Replacing car seats

If you are ever in a car accident, even a minor one, it is essential that you replace your baby's car seat – in a survey by Norwich Union (now Aviva) nearly half of parents said that they wouldn't bother forking out £100 to replace the car seat after an accident. And yet these seats can be weakened or damaged, which means that they don't offer the same protection – and the damage isn't always apparent. For the same reason you should never use second-hand car seats – it is illegal to sell them. Don't be tempted to borrow them from friends.

WHEN TO SEE A DOCTOR

Undescended testes

In the womb, baby boys' testes form in the abdomen then descend into the scrotal sac at around week 36 of pregnancy. But in around 3 per cent of boys this doesn't happen and the testes don't descend fully, sometimes remaining in the abdomen – in premature babies this is more common, affecting about 30 per cent of boys. Visually, boys with this condition look similar to boys without it, although if you look closely you will notice that their sacs are empty.

Undescended testes isn't a serious condition because it doesn't cause pain or problems urinating and it generally rights itself without intervention – the testes will simply descend of their own accord. By the age of three months, the problem will have resolved itself in two-thirds of boys born with the condition because their testes will descend naturally. For the remaining third, it's a waiting game because there's still a good chance that the problem will sort itself out. Note that you are most likely to see the testes in the scrotal sac when your son is in a warm bath, and that they will retract into the groin when he is cold or sometimes if the testes are touched. It can be quite difficult to see whether a baby's testes have descended, so speak to a health professional if you are worried.

If your son's testes haven't descended by the time he is six months old, ask your doctor for a referral to a paediatric surgeon because he will need to have a minor operation between the ages of one and two to correct the condition. This is necessary because the testes can become too warm in the abdomen and this can affect sperm production and fertility later on. It would also increase his risk of testicular cancer – partly because the testes would be more susceptible to cancer as they are warmer in the abdomen, and also because it isn't possible to check for testicular cancer manually if the testes haven't descended.

WHAT'S HAPPENING TO MUM

Melanin production increases during pregnancy, which may have left you with a dark line from your belly button to your pubic bone. You may also have noticed that any freckles or moles became darker, and that your face looked tanned. By now this discoloration will have begun to fade although it can take over six months for it to disappear completely.

PLANNING AHEAD
Swimming lessons

If you want to teach your baby to swim, then enrol him for baby swimming lessons because he'll be able to use a public pool once he's completed his five-in-one vaccination programme at around week 16 (see page 133). You can either take him to a mum and baby group that teaches babies to enjoy the water with lots of songs and games, or find something a little more serious that trains your baby to swim underwater with the aim of him saving himself should he ever accidentally fall into water. Newborns have an innate ability to propel themselves along underwater, but your baby loses this at about four months. However, it's still possible to teach your baby to swim underwater and most babies enjoy swimming classes.

Be aware that chlorine can be drying, which isn't ideal if your baby has eczema – put lots of emollient on after his swim and be prepared to give up the classes if his skin seems to get noticeably worse. For class details, ask at your local pool, and also try schools in your area that have a swimming pool – they often rent them out for baby and toddler lessons.

week 15

If your baby suddenly appears irritable and wants to be picked up all the time, he could be teething. It's quite common for teeth to start causing pain from around now, even if they don't actually come through for another few months. You'll notice that as soon as the teeth break through the gums the pain stops, and that your baby becomes most distressed in the few hours before the tooth 'pops'.

Look out for dribbling, biting, red gums, red cheeks, disturbed sleep and ear rubbing. All of these can be signs that teeth are coming, and the first ones to appear are usually the two lower incisors at the front of the mouth. Don't be afraid to give your baby regular doses of baby paracetamol such as Calpol if teething seems to be making him miserable – giving it to him every night for a couple of weeks to help him sleep won't harm him if you keep to the recommended dose. And if Calpol cheers him up, it indicates that he was genuinely in pain. Cooled teething rings and anaesthetic gels such as Bonjela also give relief, and some mums swear by homeopathic remedies.

Another side effect of teething is that excessive dribbling can irritate the skin around the mouth and chin. Don't rub your baby's chin as this triggers saliva production, but instead dab the dribble away gently – you could also apply Aqueous Cream (from pharmacists) if the skin looks sore. The extra saliva is also thought to loosen the bowels, but take care that you don't overlook a genuine case of diarrhoea by dismissing it as teething. Some mums are convinced that whenever their baby gets a new tooth, nappy rash develops but there's no medical explanation so it could just be coincidence.

As for when your baby will get his teeth, the average age is six months, but there are no rules – some babies are born with teeth and some don't get any until they are a year old. But between four and nine months is usual for a first tooth to appear.

SLEEP

Total sleep required: 14–16 hours a day
Pattern: aim for your baby to have at least five hours of uninterrupted sleep at night, for him to go to bed early, and to have three daytime naps

This week, you might want to start thinking about your baby's daytime napping pattern. In week six we explained that your baby was too young to follow a very defined napping pattern (see page 112), but now he's definitely old enough to have set nap times. The advantage of organising his daytime naps is that it will help him to sleep better at night because he won't become overtired and fractious and unable to calm down. Also, learning to settle himself for a nap is good practice for being able to settle himself more easily at night.

The downside of having scheduled nap times is that you lose flexibility – when babies are first born you can pop them in a sling or pram and they will simply sleep when they need to and you don't have to plan your day with too much precision. But as they get older babies don't drop off quite so easily during the day and you'll find yourself jiggling the pram as your baby howls in a supermarket, or pushing your screaming baby round the block to get him off to sleep while your friends wait in a café.

If you have a rough idea of when your baby is due for his daytime sleeps, it will make it easier to settle him during the day and hopefully limit any overtired crying. Ideally, he should nap in his cot because this will help him to sleep soundly in his cot at night. But realistically, you are bound to be out and about for some of your baby's daytime naps. So compromise by letting your baby have at least one of his naps in his cot. What you're aiming for is that your baby has about half of his daytime sleeps at a set time in his cot by the time he is six months old as this will help your baby sleep through the night.

What time your baby should nap

At this age your baby will probably need three naps a day. The first will begin as early as 90 minutes after he wakes in the morning and will probably last for about half an hour. Then he'll have a longer lunchtime nap – it's a good idea to put him in his cot for this nap and encourage him to sleep for a couple of hours. This is his main nap of the day which he will continue to need until he is about three – so put the effort in now to get this napping habit well established because it will give you a guaranteed daily breathing space for the next three years.

His final nap will be late in the afternoon, perhaps at about 4.30pm, and will probably last about 30 minutes. This is the first nap that your baby will drop, probably when he is about five months old, but in the meantime, ensure that this nap ends at least two hours before bedtime so as not to disrupt your baby's night sleep.

FEEDING

Total milk required: 720–1200 ml/24–40 oz a day
(up to 240 ml/8 oz per feed)
Pattern: 5–8 feeds a day

If your baby is teething, it can make sucking very painful and his gums will tingle. You'll notice that he seems hungry but then pulls away from the nipple or teat, shaking his head and crying with pain.

He'll be willing enough to continue the feed but once again he'll find it too uncomfortable to continue. This is different from appetite loss, which can occur if your baby is unwell, because then your baby won't show much interest in milk in the first place.

You can use a teat with a bigger hole if your baby is bottle-fed, or even try him on a cup as this puts less pressure on the gums because it doesn't require as much suction. Giving him baby paracetamol, such as Calpol, 15 minutes before a feed will also help. If you opt for Calpol, then watch the dose and be aware that you won't be able to administer pain relief with every feed.

WASHING

Think about introducing some rituals into bathtime, such as particular songs to wash your baby's hair, or perhaps a rhyme to get out of the bath. This not only makes bathtime fun, but also becomes part of his end of the day winding down and bedtime routine, which will become more important as your baby gets older. He'll find these babyhood rhymes and songs particularly comforting as he becomes a toddler.

From now on very little changes as far as washing is concerned so we'll no longer be covering it as a separate section. The exception is when your baby starts on solids so we've included a final washing section in week 17.

DEVELOPMENT AND PLAYING

Some babies will roll over for the first time around now. They'll move from their front to their back when they happen to lift their head to see what is going on and end up tipping themselves on to their backs. Your baby will be surprised but pleased the first time this happens so give him lots of praise.

Carpets and cots are the best places for your baby to practise his rolling skills as these are soft but also give some grip, but it will take him at least another week before he's able to roll on to his back with ease. As for rolling from his back to his tummy, this requires more strength so may not happen for another month or so. When it does, your baby may choose to sleep on his front sometimes. This is fine and you don't need to worry too much about cot death because your baby is well able to roll on to his back again with ease.

If you've ever tried playing peekaboo with your baby, you probably haven't had a great response. While he's delighted to see your face, you'll find that as soon as you hide behind your hands his face goes blank and he forgets that you were ever there in the first place. This is because he's still too young to have developed what is known as 'object permanence' – which means that if he can't see something then as far as he's concerned it doesn't exist. But once you remove your hands and your baby sees your face again, he'll be excited because his recognition skills are developed and he knows who you are. Your baby won't develop object permanence until he's around six months and until then he lives in a magical world where objects and people simply appear and disappear before his eyes.

! SAFETY TIP OF THE WEEK !
Don't leave your baby seat on the bed

Avoid putting baby seats or car seats on tables or beds as they can topple off when your baby wriggles. These should only ever be placed on the floor or in cars. This is particularly important from now onwards because your baby is quite wriggly so likely to move quite vigorously in his seat. And, of course, NEVER leave him unattended on a bed or sofa.

WHEN TO SEE A DOCTOR

Conjunctivitis

Eye infections can often occur when your baby has a cold if the virus happens to affect his eyes. He may also get conjunctivitis if he comes into contact with toddlers because there's a good chance that children will touch his eyes out of curiosity. Symptoms include sticky eyes in the morning, and also the inside of his lower eyelids will be bright red. To begin with, your baby may have an infection in just one eye but it is very likely to spread to the other eye.

Conjunctivitis isn't usually serious but can cause discomfort. The infection generally lasts for a few days if it is bacterial, in which case it can be treated with antibiotic ointment from your GP. If it is a viral infection, it may take a couple of weeks to clear up by itself.

Conjunctivitis is often linked with a cold, and if that's the case it will clear up as the cold disappears. Although conjunctivitis goes away on its own, do see a doctor if your baby's eyes look sore for longer than 24 hours.

It's impossible to say whether the infection is viral or bacterial without taking a swab so most GPs prescribe antibiotic ointment as a fail-safe. Unlike oral antibiotics, there isn't a problem with using antibiotic eye ointments quite freely. To remove morning stickiness, wash your baby's eyes with cotton wool soaked in cooled, boiled water, using a separate piece of cotton wool for each eye to reduce cross infection. You should also wash your baby's towel each day while he's infected, and not let anyone else in the family use it.

WHAT'S HAPPENING TO MUM

Pregnancy makes your hair thicker because growth slows and old hair stops falling out. But hair growth resumes around now and the old hair will begin to fall out rapidly. Expect to see blocked plugholes, and hair all over your pillow for the next few months – which can be alarming initially but is nothing to worry about. If you're breast-feeding, you may have to wait until you cut down on nursing before you experience hair loss. Don't worry about hair loss because you won't end up with thinner hair.

You may want to increase your iron intake (see page 157) because being anaemic can sometimes cause thinning hair.

PLANNING AHEAD
Buy a teething kit

Stock up on teething rings that can be put in the freezer, tubes of numbing gel such as Bonjela, and baby paracetamol such as Calpol. Teething pain always gets worse at night when your baby is lying down as this makes the gums throb more, so it's a good idea to have some soothers to hand.

week 16

From this week onwards you could, theoretically, get a good night's sleep. This is because once your baby is four months old and weighs 7.3 kg/16 lb or more, he has the capacity to go for eight hours without feeding. If you're lucky enough to have a baby who starts sleeping through around now, then congratulations. But do bear in mind that it's quite common for babies to regress and start waking in the night again, so keep working on your baby's good sleep habits such as having a regular bedtime and allowing him to settle himself with no help from you.

If your baby is nowhere near sleeping through the night then console yourself with the fact that you are in the majority – less than a quarter of all babies in the UK sleep through the night by the age of 10 months according to the Economic and Social Research Council.

At 16 weeks a lot of parents blame hunger for their baby's limited sleep and say that their child needs to be on solids before he can go through the night. But there's no evidence that eating solids extends sleep and babies are definitely able to sleep for eight hours on formula or breast milk alone.

The other event to occur this week is your baby's third batch of immunisations. If for some reason they have been delayed because your baby had a cold or you couldn't get the appointment that you wanted, don't worry because the delay won't reduce the effectiveness of the vaccines in any way. Just book another appointment soon.

SLEEP

Total sleep required: *14–16 hours a day*
Pattern: *aim for your baby to have eight hours of uninterrupted sleep at night, for him to go to bed early, and to have three daytime naps*

Some babies will be sleeping for up to eight hours, uninterrupted, at night by now. If your baby isn't yet sleeping well at night then you are no doubt disappointed, not to mention exhausted. While there are no quick fixes for teaching babies to sleep through the night, there are plenty of steps you can take – and getting him into a good napping pattern is one of them.

Last week we explained how teaching your baby to settle himself at nap time (see page 200) will help him learn to settle himself throughout the night. What you're aiming for is to be able to put your baby down in his cot, leave him to settle himself after about five minutes and for him to then sleep soundly for an hour or two. This will take quite a lot of time and patience, but one advantage of 'working' on his day sleeps is that you'll have more energy and patience than trying to sleep train your baby in the middle of the night.

Teaching your baby good napping habits

1. Observe your baby for signs of tiredness
As soon as your baby rubs his eyes, seems fractious, less energetic or active, then it's nap time. You'll have to put him down for a sleep quite quickly because his sleep window can be quite narrow during the day before he gets another burst of energy. Also his nap time can change slightly depending on his previous night's sleep and how active he's been during the morning. But once you've got the napping

habit established, your baby will feel tired at around the same time each day.

2. Introduce a napping routine

Just like at bedtime, your baby will need a clear sign that it's time to go to sleep. You can keep this short and simple, perhaps a drink of milk, then pop him into his sleeping bag before putting him down.

3. Soothe your baby to sleep

Ideally your baby will settle himself to sleep, but at this age he's likely to need a bit of help getting to sleep for his daytime nap. As always, the less you do the better, so avoid too much rocking and stick to a simple technique such as rubbing his tummy while you stand next to his cot, or just holding him still in your arms.

4. What to do if he cries

It's likely that your baby will protest and tell you that he doesn't want to go to sleep. Go through a checklist to ensure that he's fed, has a clean nappy, that he's ready for a sleep because he's been awake for more than two hours, and that he isn't ill or in pain. Then you can be pretty sure that your baby's tearful protest is because he is in fact tired and needs to sleep. Stay calm while he cries and don't falter by chopping and changing your chosen soothing technique. It may help you to wear ear plugs to take the intensity out of his crying, and also to time his tears because at this age they probably won't go on for much longer than about 15 minutes. You will notice that your baby's crying pattern gradually switches from constant crying with the occasional pause, to a constant pause with the occasional cry. And he may well cry most vigorously for 5–10 minutes. Try to remain calm and confident, remind yourself that he needs to go to sleep and that as his mother you are teaching him the important skill of self-soothing. If you possibly can, resist resorting to feeding him to sleep.

5. Extend your baby's nap time

Your baby is likely to wake after just 40 minutes because this is the length of his sleep cycle. If you are on hand at this time to gently sshh him and rub his tummy he may well go off to sleep again and eventually learn to re-settle himself.

FEEDING

Total milk required: 720–1200 ml/24–40 oz a day
(up to 240 ml/8 oz per feed)
Pattern: 5–7 feeds a day

The weaning debate is a complex one, which we shall cover in detail in week 17 (see pages 214 and 217) and you shouldn't give your baby solids before next week.

DEVELOPMENT AND PLAYING

If your baby is happy spending time on his tummy and has done so regularly over the last few months, then he will be well practised in pushing his chest off the floor. By now he'll be able to push himself up and rest on his forearms for a couple of minutes while he has a good look around. This strengthens his arm and trunk muscles in preparation for crawling at about seven months.

Your baby will 'find' his hands this week and will start sucking and playing with them. If you've been swaddling your baby then you can leave his hands free from now onwards so that he can suck his hands as he comforts himself to sleep. Learning to self-soothe is an important step in being able to sleep for hours without needing help from mum. Your baby's hands will also provide plenty of entertainment as he studies them and pulls at his fingers.

WHEN TO SEE A DOCTOR

Bronchiolitis

Bronchiolitis is a viral infection that babies can catch between September and April, and is a common illness which affects up to 90 per cent of children before they are aged two. Once your child has developed an immunity to the respiratory syncytial virus, RSV, he is unlikely to get bronchiolitis again.

Bronchiolitis begins with a cold that lasts about four days, before developing into a dry rasping cough for a few days. This is usually followed by a wet chesty cough which goes on for another 10 days or so as the bronchioles (smaller breathing tubes) in the lungs are affected by the virus. Your baby may develop a fever and feel unwell with a heavy cold and cough. Most babies will fight the virus off by themselves and parents aren't even aware that their baby had bronchiolitis but assume he had a heavy cold.

To diagnose bronchiolitis the nurse takes a phlegm sample by sticking a tube gently and briefly up your baby's nose. Another giveaway that your baby had bronchiolitis is that some babies go on to develop a post-bronchiolitis cough which can last up to eight weeks – during this time your baby should feel well, feed well and put on weight.

When bronchiolitis gets serious

Some babies with bronchiolitis are particularly hard hit and need to be admitted to hospital. So seek medical help if your baby exhibits any of the following:

- Feeding poorly – this is worse than just having a blocked nose and finding it more difficult to feed than normal – only worry if your baby is barely drinking any milk at all.
- He seems miserable and worn out – you'll know if your baby is not his usual self.
- Reduced urine – this ties in with poor feeding. If your baby has a completely dry nappy for longer than five hours then see a doctor.
- Apnoea – this is when your baby stops breathing for 10 seconds or more, and it can happen while he is both awake or asleep. It's normal for babies to have short pauses when breathing and to breathe erratically. If your baby has apnoea then get medical help.
- Struggling to breathe – being bunged up and snuffly is normal and nothing to worry about, but if your baby seems to be fighting for breath this is a problem and it will be obvious that something is wrong. Take him to your hospital's Emergency Department.
- Blue lips or tongue – this means that your baby is finding it hard to breathe and has become short of oxygen. Blue lips can sometimes just mean that he is very cold. If he's not cold then take him to your hospital's Emergency Department.

WHAT'S HAPPENING TO MUM

You'll probably find that you feel more stressed now that you are a mum. Gone are the days when you could slob around doing nothing at the weekend after a busy week, or have a massive lie-in to make up for a big night. These days you're on duty 24/7 – even when your baby is fast asleep, you're still responsible for him.

There's no getting away from the fact that being a parent is hard work which can take its toll on your stress levels. So it's essential that you introduce some coping strategies because things aren't going to change very much for quite a while.

Think about what you did to relax before you had children. Even if you used to exercise most mornings, or go out most nights – just doing these things as little as once a fortnight will make a difference. Persuade your partner to take your baby out in the buggy for an hour – there's something instantly relaxing about having your home to yourself for a while.

Post-natal depression (PND) can occur any time in the first year but it is most likely to develop when your baby is between four and six months old, so from around now. It may come on suddenly or begin very gradually, even if everyone thinks you are 'coping' extremely well.

PND can have many symptoms including thinking that life has become a long grey tunnel, or perhaps you feel tearful, irritable, anxious, guilty, lethargic, or worried that you're not a good mum.

Speak to your health visitor or GP. PND was covered in week four and week nine (see pages 93 and 157). You can also get details from www.mind.org.uk

PLANNING AHEAD
Buy equipment for solids

If you're intending to start your baby on solids over the next few weeks, you will need to buy the following:

- a plastic weaning spoon (these are slim and soft and designed to be slipped into babies' mouths)
- bibs
- baby rice – this comes dried and you mix it with breast milk or formula. If you're breastfeeding then you can either express milk to mix with the baby rice or use formula milk.

You will be able to buy all this from your pharmacist.

week 17

If you've been thinking about starting your baby on solids, this week is the very earliest that you should begin – and if your baby was premature then you should wait until 17 weeks after his due date. Giving your baby solids earlier than this could put a strain on his digestive system and kidneys.

Current advice is to wait until six months before giving your baby solids, but weaning advice is forever changing. Previous generations raced to get their infants eating baby food, sometimes at just a month old – if a baby took to solids it was thought to show how quickly he was developing. Then it was recommended that mothers weaned their babies between four and six months, but this advice was followed by recommendations from the World Health Organisation that stated mothers should exclusively breastfeed or bottle-feed for six months before introducing solids.

The Department of Health still recommends waiting until six months, but the latest scientific opinion from the European Food Safety Authority states that it is safe to begin solids while still breast-feeding, at any time between four and six months.

Confused? Then you're certainly not alone. But there's a lot of research going on in this area and guidelines will no doubt settle and become clearer in the coming years. But in the meantime, we suggest aiming to give your baby his first solids by the time he's six months, but not fretting or feeling guilty if you decide to wean a bit earlier. It's essential not to delay weaning until after six months because this can lead to problems with growth, iron deficiency and learning to chew.

The big advantage of waiting until six months is that by this age, your baby will be able to eat most foods and will also be old enough to try finger foods. It is certainly easier to wean a six-month-old baby than a four-month-old. And you'll be able to try baby-led weaning which is when babies always feed themselves – this isn't appropriate for younger babies because they are not physically developed enough to cope with finger foods.

SLEEP

Total sleep required: 14–16 hours a day
Pattern: aim for your baby to have eight hours of uninterrupted sleep at night, for him to go to bed early, and to have three daytime naps

Continuing the all-consuming topic of teaching your baby to sleep through the night, we look this week at how to drop his night feeds. If your baby weighs 7.3 kg/16 lb or more, then he is physically capable of sleeping for eight hours without a feed. But the reality is likely to be a different story. Most babies of this age will naturally wake up four times during the night – so if you put your baby to bed at 7pm, there's a good chance that he'll wake at about 8 or 9pm, then again at about midnight, then probably between 2 and 3am, and finally very early in the morning at about 5am.

Ideally your baby will drop off to sleep again easily and without fuss for at least three of these awakenings and perhaps want food for the fourth. But your baby may demand food for all four awakenings, and if he's getting fed four times a night he will feel genuinely hungry at these times, even though he's now physically capable of going for a decent length of time without food. So aim to cut these feeds out one by one until your baby is waking just once a night. Begin with the 8–9pm feed which is the easiest to drop as your baby is unlikely to be hungry so soon after his bedtime feed. Give your baby slightly less milk at this feed so that he gradually becomes accustomed to not eating at this time. If you're bottle-feeding, cut the feed by 30 ml/1 oz every couple of days; if you're breastfeeding, reduce the length of the feed by two minutes every couple of days. Within a couple of weeks your baby will hopefully have dropped this feed and will no longer be waking.

There's another way of dropping feeds and that is to feed your baby later than he demands. So if he always wakes at 8pm, don't feed him until 9pm – keep delaying until he's not waking up until midnight, when he was due for his second feed of the night anyway. Your baby is likely to get upset when you don't feed him on demand but you can comfort him in other ways, perhaps just standing by the cot and stroking him. It'll take about three nights for him to get used to the new timetable. Once you've dropped the 8pm feed, you can pick another one to drop until eventually your baby won't be feeding at night.

IS YOUR BABY SLEEPING THROUGH THE NIGHT YET?

Be aware that most parents exaggerate when it comes to describing how 'good' their baby is at night – you might want to think about stretching the truth a little yourself. Friends and relatives will enquire constantly about how your baby sleeps and if you admit that he hasn't yet adopted a 'textbook' sleeping pattern, you can expect an onslaught of conflicting and confusing advice. It's not a competition or a race, and the occasional fib will certainly help you get through these tough weeks of sleep deprivation.

FEEDING

Total milk required: 720–1200 ml/24–40 oz a day (up to 240 ml/8 oz in one feed)
Pattern: 5–7 feeds, plus solids – one teaspoon of baby rice mixed with milk a day

The following signs may indicate that your baby is physically ready to eat solids. You may notice him becoming more aware of food from around now.

Signs that your baby wants solids

- He is putting things in his mouth and is interested in your food, watching closely as you eat, perhaps trying to grab at your fork or plate. This is the biggest giveaway that your baby is ready to be weaned because he is 'telling' you that he wants food.

- He is waking in the night more than he used to and demanding to be fed.
- He has started to get hungry within an hour of a feed.

IS YOUR BABY READY FOR SOLIDS?

If your baby is showing some of the above signs that he's getting hungrier, then he's probably nearly ready to go on to solids. But do check the following list before you begin. This will ensure that he's physically capable of eating solid food.

- Your baby has doubled his birth weight, which is important because he won't put weight on as quickly once he starts on solids. Puréed carrot and baby rice are more filling than milk, so your baby will feel satisfied more easily on solids and take in fewer calories.
- He can hold his head steadily and sit up well when supported.
- There's no history of food allergy in the family – if there is, then your baby should be six months old before moving on to solids.
- He has lost his tongue-thrust reflex, which makes him automatically reject anything that enters his mouth by pushing it out with his tongue. This is a protective mechanism which you won't observe until you actually start giving your baby solids. Be

prepared to postpone solids for a few weeks if your baby appears to still have this reflex after several attempts at feeding.

If you've ticked the first three points in our checklist, you can think about giving your baby solids. If you've decided not to introduce your baby to solids just yet, then you can be confident that breast milk or formula is perfectly adequate for him until he's six months and that he's not missing out nutritionally in any way.

Weaning first step – baby rice

You can buy boxes of dried baby rice from chemists and supermarkets, which you mix with either breast milk or formula. The bland milky taste will be familiar to your baby and rice is unlikely to cause an allergic reaction, which makes it a good first food. Begin by mixing just one teaspoon of rice and follow the directions on the box to get the quantity of milk correct. The consistency should be quite liquid to begin with, like thick soup, and it doesn't have to be warmed up.

Your baby will start with one meal so choose a time that roughly coincides with either breakfast, lunch or tea when your baby usually has a milk feed. Try giving your baby his solids about 10 minutes before his milk feed is due. He'll be wide awake and hungry but not yet getting ravenous and fractious. Of course, if he's getting cranky then try giving him half or even all of his milk feed before resuming the solids.

Use a plastic baby spoon to feed your baby as this is softer and less likely to bash his gums than a metal spoon – you can buy baby spoons from chemists. Then sit your baby up, either in a baby seat or on your lap, and spoon some baby rice into his mouth. He'll probably be quite surprised and will almost certainly spit it out. But try another few spoonfuls and don't worry if your baby doesn't seem to eat anything at all – your goal is simply to get him to experience solid food in his mouth. It will be messy and a lot of the rice will end up on your baby's face as well as on the floor. By the end of the week, your baby may swallow the occasional spoonful as he gets used to moving the food from the front to the back of his mouth. But your main aim is to keep mealtimes short, fun and relaxed, so don't worry about how much he eats.

If your baby tells you that he doesn't want to eat by clamping his mouth or turning his head away, then let him skip a meal. He'll probably want to try again the next day. It may turn out that this week is too soon for your baby to be weaned. So if he doesn't get the hang of feeding at all and seems disinterested, then have the confidence to follow his wishes – pack away the baby rice and try again in a couple of weeks.

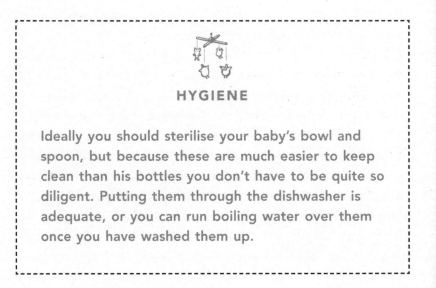

HYGIENE

Ideally you should sterilise your baby's bowl and spoon, but because these are much easier to keep clean than his bottles you don't have to be quite so diligent. Putting them through the dishwasher is adequate, or you can run boiling water over them once you have washed them up.

FOOD ALLERGIES AND INTOLERANCES

Whenever you introduce a new food to your baby, keep an eye out for signs of an allergic reaction or intolerance. If you haven't noticed any rashes, vomiting or diarrhoea within three days, the new food gets the all-clear. Don't introduce new foods at the evening feed because your baby could be up all night with indigestion, and more importantly you wouldn't necessarily notice a rash at night. If your baby reacts mildly to a new food, leave it for a few weeks before attempting to reintroduce it.

NAPPIES

Number of wet nappies over 24 hours: 4–8
Number of dirty nappies over 24 hours: 0–5

Introducing solids to your baby shouldn't result in any change in his urine output and the number of wet nappies a day shouldn't decrease. His poos may become a little firmer, and possibly slightly less frequent over the next few weeks.

WASHING

At bathtime, ensure that you wash under your baby's chin because food can get trapped in his neck creases.

DEVELOPMENT AND PLAYING

As we mentioned last week, your baby can probably push up on to his forearms by now when he's lying on his tummy, and the next step is to be able to lift his chest and legs off the floor at the same time. Again this helps your baby to strengthen his trunk muscles in preparation for crawling. In the meantime he'll enjoy waving his arms and playing 'aeroplanes'.

From now onwards, your baby will love you singing nursery rhymes to him, especially if you do the actions with him – for example 'row the boat'. Once you've repeated a song about six times your baby will start to recognise it and you'll soon have a few favourites which you'll probably keep singing together well into his toddler years.

> **! SAFETY TIP OF THE WEEK !**
> **Move hazardous objects away from your baby**
>
> Once your baby is rolling, take care not to leave anything dangerous nearby, such as plastic bags or small objects that he might try eating. Always overestimate how far your baby may roll – he's bound to surprise you.

WHEN TO SEE A DOCTOR

Heat rash (prickly heat)

This is a common rash that develops if your baby is too hot – usually during the summer because you've wrapped him up in too many layers. Your baby's sweat glands aren't yet fully developed and so he's unable to properly cool himself. Instead of 'sweating', the glands can become blocked, which leads to the inflammation known as heat rash. You'll see small pink bumps and blisters, often in the creases around the nappy, and also on your baby's trunk, face and under his arms. Your baby will probably be irritable because he feels too hot, and may have flushed cheeks.

Cool your baby down by removing some of his clothes, and if he's still flushed after an hour, give him a cool sponge bath. Offer him milk to keep him hydrated and open the windows. The rash should soon fade, but call your doctor if your baby hasn't cooled down after three hours or if he has a fever – that is a temperature higher than 38°C/100.4°F.

WHAT'S HAPPENING TO MUM

If you're breastfeeding and decide to start your baby on solids this week, you may notice that your weight loss begins to slow down over the next couple of months. This is because you won't be producing as much breast milk and therefore won't be burning so many calories.

The upside is that as you cut back on breastfeeding, you won't feel so hungry which will help you to lose your baby weight.

Some women find that it is only when they stop breastfeeding altogether that they are able to shed those last few pounds – women's bodies build up fat reserves while they are pregnant and sometimes this can't be lost while you are breastfeeding.

PLANNING AHEAD
Book a weekend away

By now you'll be proficient at looking after your baby – feeding and changing his nappies on autopilot. He'll hopefully be sleeping better at night which will mean you have a bit more energy.

This is a relatively easy stage before you have to start weaning your baby in the coming weeks and months, and also before he becomes mobile – usually from around six months.

We suggest that you make the most of this time and book a weekend away, go on a long train journey to visit friends or relatives, or go on holiday. It's also a good time to book hair and dental appointments, and even go shoe shopping!

Babies love anything different and your baby will be fascinated by trains, buses, automatic doors, new faces, all of which will seem like a big adventure. Make the most of the fact that he's happy to stay in his buggy because he can't yet move, and also that you're not fussing about with jars and purees as he's still on milk only. If you choose to fly he'll travel free and he'll happily drink milk at take-off to help with his ears.

week 18

Teaching your baby to eat is an exciting time and this week we move on from baby rice and introduce two new foods so that he can experience fresh tastes. Feeding your baby can, however, be fraught with anxiety and most mums worry that their child isn't eating enough – or later that he isn't eating healthily enough. Ironically, worrying is about the worst thing you can do when it comes to feeding your baby because he'll pick up on your stress and this can reduce how much he eats. Be reassured by the fact that if there's food on offer, your baby won't go short even if he's off his food for a day or so.

As for a healthy diet, now's the time to instil good habits because your baby will happily taste everything that you spoon into his mouth. If over the next few months you introduce him to as wide a menu as possible, he'll be less fussy when he's older and more likely to accept vegetables rather than sticking stubbornly to chicken nuggets.

The key message with weaning is to relax, be gentle and teach by example. So whenever you feel anxious about what your child is or isn't eating, turn your attention to your own diet. If you're eating five portions of fresh fruit and vegetables a day, plus lots of home-cooked dishes, your child will end up eating a similar diet.

SLEEP

Total sleep required: 14–16 hours a day
*Pattern: aim for your baby to have eight hours of
uninterrupted sleep at night, for him to go to bed early, and
to have three daytime naps*

If your baby has been sleeping in your bed (see page 96), then you
may want to think about breaking this habit before he becomes too
used to the luxury of cuddling up with mum and dad at night. Some
parents love sharing their beds with their babies and you may decide
to let nature dictate when your baby gets his own cot or bed. There's
nothing wrong with your baby remaining in your bed for a few years
as long as everyone's happy with the arrangement and this works for
your family. But most parents want their own bed back much sooner
than this, in which case it's time to start teaching your baby to sleep
in his own cot. The most likely scenario is that your baby has his
own cot and comes into your bed at some stage during the night
when he wakes for a feed.

This is quite an easy pattern to break because your baby is used to
going off to sleep by himself. Begin by staying awake when you feed
him in the night so that you can put him back in his cot afterwards.
It may take a bit of time to settle him back into his own bed – not
easy when you're exhausted in the middle of the night. But it's worth
the effort now because if you leave it, you'll find that your baby
becomes ever more difficult to persuade as he gets older.

Some babies won't go to sleep in a cot at all but will only sleep in
their parents' bed – this means that you have to lie down with your
baby for him to nod off. If you're in this situation and not happy
about it, then it's time to go back to some basic sleep-training techniques and teach your baby to settle himself. Refer to earlier chapters,
beginning in week three (see page 63), for a step by step guide to
teaching your baby to get to sleep by himself.

FEEDING

*Total milk required: 720–1200 ml/24–40 oz a day
(up to 240 ml/8 oz per feed)*
*Pattern: 5–7 feeds, plus solids – two teaspoons of baby rice mixed
with milk, plus a little puréed carrot or pear purée twice a day*

Weaning – puréed carrot and pear

Hopefully your baby swallowed a little baby rice last week, in which
case you can proceed with weaning him and move on to puréed
carrot. Otherwise, persevere for another couple of days with the rice
and if you don't see an improvement, abandon weaning for the
moment and try again in a few weeks.

Your goal this week is to introduce your baby to new tastes which
he will probably enjoy – again you don't have to worry if he doesn't
actually eat very much because milk is still his main food source.
Carrots are a good early food because they are naturally sweet,
which babies like, and also unlikely to cause an allergic reaction.
Boil some up until very soft – if you use fresh carrots then make sure
that you peel them, or you can use frozen for convenience. Mash
the boiled carrots with a fork or potato masher then push them
through a sieve so that you have a very smooth mixture – you can
also use a food processor, blender or a mouli (you grind the food
by hand). Mix one or two teaspoons of carrot with some formula
or breast milk until it is the consistency of thick soup – you can
mix in a little baby rice if you want to. However, you don't have
to mix the carrot with anything at all – the only reason for doing
so is that it keeps the taste familiar, bulks it out and also gives you
control over the consistency as you balance the amount of milk
and rice that you add. Offer your baby as much carrot as he wants
– he won't over-eat at this age. You can continue to use baby rice
throughout the weaning programme whenever you want to bulk a
purée out. The purée should never be kept once you've added milk,
but you can store puréed carrot without added milk in the fridge

for 24 hours. You can also freeze the puréed carrot without added milk in ice-cube trays – you'll need about one cube per meal at this stage (see page 234).

If your baby shows no adverse reaction to carrot after three days, you can offer him puréed pear which you peel, boil, mash and sieve just as you did with the carrots. You now have three choices for your baby – rice, carrot and pear. As your baby becomes more competent at swallowing food over the next few weeks, you can make the consistency a little thicker by adding baby rice – make the mixture thick enough so that you can tilt the spoon slightly without it falling off.

DEVELOPMENT AND PLAYING

About now you will notice that your baby is better at picking things up because he has learnt to use his thumb separately to his four fingers – this allows him to use his hands like a claw giving him more precision. He won't be able to pick up tiny objects with his thumb and index finger until he is eight months old.

Although your baby can't sit up by himself yet, if you hold him by his hands in the sitting position you will find that instead of his back being completely rounded like a newborn, the upper part of his back is now strong and upright. He has also gained strength in his neck muscles, which allows him to hold his head steady. Your baby won't be able to sit up unsupported until he is at least six months, and even then he'll be very wobbly.

!SAFETY TIP OF THE WEEK!
Avoid baby walkers

Don't put your baby in a baby walker – a plastic-framed seat on wheels that babies can 'walk' around in. These give babies mobility that is way above their own motion skills at this age, and this is dangerous and leads to high numbers of accidents, such as reaching for knives or falling down stairs.

WHEN TO SEE A DOCTOR

Vomiting

For the first few months your baby would have brought up milk every now and again, perhaps frequently if he was a particularly 'sicky' baby. But as he gets older, vomiting can sometimes indicate something more serious. If your baby vomits as a one-off then there's no need to worry – minor infections such as a cold or sore throat can cause vomiting in babies, and excess mucus and coughing can also make your baby sick.

Should your baby vomit more than twice in 24 hours and he isn't usually a 'sicky' baby, then you should consider seeing your doctor. Vomiting accompanied by diarrhoea is likely to be gastroenteritis (a gut infection) or food poisoning in which case your baby is at risk of becoming dehydrated. You can treat him at home by giving him plenty of milk to keep his fluids up. You can also use a re-hydration mixture such as Dioralyte to replace lost salts and fluids – this is available over the counter from chemists – and give your baby weak orange or blackcurrant squash because the sugar helps absorption and increases fluid uptake.

If your baby passes less urine than usual, or you don't see a wet nappy for over six hours, then take him to the doctor because dehydration in babies is extremely dangerous. Another sign of dehydration is cool fingers and toes. Your doctor will probably prescribe Dioralyte and may ask for a stool sample to identify the bug causing the tummy upset.

Sometimes vomiting can indicate a serious problem, for instance if there's blood in your baby's vomit and you are sure that this isn't because of breastfeeding and bleeding nipples. Blood in vomit always needs investigating and you should take your baby to your hospital's Emergency Department. You should also take him to hospital if his vomit is bright green or yellow, which can happen if there is a bowel obstruction, if he's eaten something poisonous, or if he's sick after a fall or a minor bump to his head.

Other illnesses that can cause your baby to vomit include a urinary tract infection (see page 251) and meningitis (see page 163). It's crucial to keep a close eye on your baby should he vomit unexpectedly because it could be a warning sign of something serious.

WHAT'S HAPPENING TO MUM

Although your baby is still only four months old, it's time to think about childcare if you're planning to go back to work. A lot of mums will already have made plans, or even have gone back to work. But if you've not yet got yourself organised there's no need to worry as plenty of women manage to find excellent childcare in the last couple of months of their maternity leave. Start asking around as you still have time to interview childminders and nannies, and to visit nurseries.

PLANNING AHEAD
Equipment for purées

Go shopping so that you can stock up on home-made frozen purées for your baby – cooking and freezing in bulk will ultimately mean less work. You'll need a blender or food processor to grind up large quantities – hand-held blenders cost less than £15 from shops such as Argos. You'll also need flexible ice-cube trays to freeze the purées, plus freezer bags to store the frozen cubes of food.

You might have considered giving your baby jars of ready-made food having tired of boiling, grinding and freezing miniature cubes of purée. And surprisingly, there's not much wrong with using jars – a lot of jars use organic ingredients these days that babies love; they're also convenient and you can be sure that they were prepared in spotless kitchens. If you are out with your baby then jars actually make more sense because transporting home-made food poses hygiene problems, particularly in the heat of summer. The downside is the expense as it's definitely cheaper to make your own food, particularly at this age when you will be throwing most of the jar away as it can't be kept for longer than 24 hours once opened.

You should also consider the negative environmental effect, and the fact that the ingredients in jars won't be as fresh. Nutritionally, jars aren't as good as home-made food as they contain a high percentage of water and therefore have fewer nutrients and calories. Once your baby starts eating meat at six months, bear in mind that jars actually contain very little meat, and that organic jars aren't fortified with iron – so it's better to choose non-organic jars after six months.

Finally, jars may taste blander than home-cooked food, which can make it harder for your baby to adjust to family meals when he's older. Nothing beats home-made food but if you do opt for jars, even just sometimes, there's no need to feel guilty because you won't be doing your child any harm, particularly at this very early weaning stage when babies get most of their nutrients and calories from milk rather than solid food.

SLEEP

Total sleep required: 14–16 hours a day
Pattern: aim for your baby to have eight hours of uninterrupted sleep at night, for him to go to bed early, and to have three daytime naps

Illness

By now your baby should have established some sort of sleep pattern if you've put the time in teaching him to settle himself back to sleep. But this can get disrupted in a few days if he becomes ill or starts teething.

You'll almost certainly realise that your baby isn't himself and that his night-time crying has changed from being overtired, annoyed or hungry to being miserable and in pain – such cries are usually higher in pitch. The rule for sick babies and children is that there are no rules. So if you've been trying to establish good sleep habits you can forget all this while your baby is ill. Give him as much comfort and milk during the night as he needs – it can actually be dangerous leaving an unwell baby to cry because his temperature could soar and you wouldn't realise if he needed medical help.

The only part of the sleep programme that you can stick to when your baby is sick is bedtime. Try to put him to bed at his normal time because this is when he's programmed to feel sleepy. Also he'll find his bedtime routine comforting, which will help to soothe him if he's feeling unwell. So if you think your baby is unwell, abandon all the sleep-training rules – feed him when he wants, let him into the bed with you if that's what he's used to, and soothe him back to sleep.

When your baby is better you'll have to remind him about good sleeping habits and re-teach him to settle himself. But he'll learn much quicker second time round, especially if his good sleep habits were already well established and he doesn't get ill for more than a few days.

FEEDING

Total milk required: 600–1200 ml/20–40 oz a day
(up to 240 ml/8 oz per feed)
Pattern: 4–6 feeds, plus solids – two cubes of purée twice a day
Weaning: some easy-to-digest fruit and vegetable purées: puréed squash, pumpkin, apple and parsnip
Weaning list so far: baby rice, carrot and pear

Continue to build up your baby's menu this week, introducing any of the new foods from the above list every few days. If your baby is enjoying his food, you can start giving him two meals a day from around now.

Freezing and storing

Now that you're in the swing of making purées for your baby, cook in bulk to save time. Boil and blend large quantities of vegetables, then scoop the purée into flexible ice-cube trays. Keep the trays covered by placing them in freezer bags, then once they are cool, put them in the freezer. Putting warm food in the freezer may defrost other food. When the cubes have frozen, pop them out into plastic bags which you can label, date, seal and store in the freezer for up to six weeks.

To defrost the cubes, microwave straight from frozen – allow a minute on full power for three cubes, stir and then microwave again for 30 seconds. The idea is to heat the purée to boiling all the way through. Stir thoroughly to avoid hot spots and allow enough cooling time – remember that babies' mouths are very sensitive to heat. You can also boil up the frozen cubes in a saucepan, or leave them over-night to defrost in the fridge before boiling them. It's important to boil all frozen food thoroughly then to eat it as soon as possible to minimise the risk of food poisoning.

Before serving, taste the food yourself to check the temperature and let your baby see you eating it because sharing food is the most natural way of encouraging him to eat. Your baby is unlikely to finish his 'meal', but don't try and save his leftovers – you need to be extremely hygienic as babies are very susceptible to food poisoning. So throw away his uneaten food, or better still eat it yourself – you'll benefit from eating extra vegetables and your baby will see that his food is delicious enough for mum to eat too.

Drinks

Milk

As your baby learns to eat more solid food, he may want slightly less milk and will probably drop a feed. However, milk remains his main food and source of nutrients until he is at least six months old.

Water

You can offer your baby boiled, cooled water from a baby cup at all his meals – cups with soft spouts work well at this age, although you may have to experiment to see which type of cup your baby prefers. Remember that some babies don't take to a cup until they are six months or older, so be patient.

Your baby probably won't like water at first because it isn't sweet, but persevere. Have a few sips yourself, make drinking from a cup into a game, and don't expect your baby to want any water himself until it's been offered at least 20 times. Even then he will only want one or two sips. But keep trying because he'll drink water eventually, and in the meantime you don't need to worry about dehydration because your baby will get most of his fluid from his milk as well as from puréed fruit and vegetables.

Milk should be your baby's main drink at mealtimes until he's eating protein, at which point you can gradually cut out any milk feeds that accompany his meals and instead give him water to quench his thirst.

Juice

Don't be tempted to offer your baby fruit juice or squash, even if it is diluted. Some people may tell you that diluted fruit juice is okay, but as far as tooth care is concerned it's not because even fresh juice contains sugar, and is acidic. It will slosh around your baby's teeth as he will drink slowly from a baby cup, and is likely to cause tooth decay.

The only advantage is that your baby will take to juice more easily than water because it tastes sweet. But once he's tasted juice, you will find it almost impossible to persuade your baby to drink water. Although juice provides your child with vitamin C, it's better to encourage him to get his vitamins from fresh fruit and vegetables which won't damage his teeth.

DEVELOPMENT AND PLAYING

Your baby will start putting everything that he grabs into his mouth around now and will suck and chew objects. This is a good way for your baby to explore new objects because his mouth is more sensitive to touch than his fingers.

Now that your baby is good at grabbing toys, he will find a mobile above his cot frustrating because he'll be desperate to touch it. A toy that attaches to the side of his cot is more appropriate because he can actually play with this. You can buy all sorts of brightly coloured animals with Velcro fastenings – but you might want to take these away at bedtime and limit them to the morning when it's time for your baby to wake up.

Morning toys in the cot are a great way of persuading your baby to let mum and dad have an extra five minutes in bed. After his early feed, you can pop your baby back in his bed with a few special toys that he only sees in the morning, and over the next few months you'll find that he's happy to spend longer and longer playing by himself in his cot.

WHEN TO SEE A DOCTOR

Ear infection

Ear tugging and head shaking both suggest that one or both of your baby's ears hurt. He may also find sucking painful and if he has a particularly severe ear infection he could scream for several hours and not want to be put down – partly because he wants comfort and also because ear pain is worse when lying down. Note that he may show similar symptoms with teething, so look out for signs of teeth about to push through the gums.

Ear infections often occur on about day four of a cold because mucus blocks the Eustachian tubes which drain the ear via the back of the throat. This means that fluid can't drain away and so fluid in the ear can become infected and the inner ear becomes inflamed.

If you suspect ear pain and your baby has a fever then take him to the doctor, who will be able to confirm an ear infection and perhaps prescribe antibiotics. Mild ear pain and no fever can be treated at home with baby paracetamol such as Calpol, but go and see your doctor if your baby is still unwell after a couple of days. Teething can also cause ear pain, and again this can be treated with baby painkillers.

Sometimes an ear infection causes the ear drum to break and yellow or white pus to drain out, usually on to your baby's bed. When this happens, it instantly relieves pain and the ear drum heals within days – you won't need to see your doctor because once the ear drum has burst the infection can heal. Gently wipe away any discharge with cotton wool, but never clean the inside of his ear and don't use cotton buds.

WHAT'S HAPPENING TO MUM

If you've breastfed your baby until now, you will have lowered his risk of asthma until he is six, and you will have cut his risk of getting an ear infection by half. If you're undecided about whether to continue to breastfeed or move on to formula, then bear in mind that breast-feeding until your baby is six months old further reduces his chances of getting asthma, and also means that you are less likely to get osteoporosis when you are older.

PLANNING AHEAD
Buy jars of food

Stock up on a few jars of food, even if you intend to give your baby a home-made diet. Jars are useful for emergencies – for example if you can't be there to feed your baby, it's easier for someone else to open a jar than to rummage through your freezer and fuss about defrosting puréed cubes. Jars are also useful when you go out, and are more hygienic than home-made food as they are sealed and don't need to be kept cool.

week 20

You've probably given your baby medicine by now, most likely Calpol (infant paracetamol) when he had his immunisations. But even if you've got a bottle of baby medicine sitting in your bathroom, there's a good chance that you feel wary about using it. Well don't – to deprive a baby of painkillers causes unnecessary suffering. Most parents hold back too much when it comes to giving their babies painkillers because of misconceptions about the dangers of drugs. But if you follow the dosage guidelines, and always use infant medicines, your baby will be perfectly safe. If you're ever unsure about whether your baby needs a painkiller, it's better to give him some because an unnecessary dose of Calpol won't do your baby any harm whatsoever.

You may think that giving your baby medicine too frequently will make him tolerant to it, but this isn't the case. The two common baby painkillers, paracetamol and ibuprofen, don't become any less effective with frequent use. Infant ibuprofen won't affect your baby's stomach lining (although this can be a risk in adults) because he eats too frequently to ever have a completely empty stomach, and his stomach lining is more resilient because he is younger. There's no need to be concerned about baby paracetamol causing your baby liver damage. Although this can occur in an adult overdose, babies metabolise this drug more efficiently so there's not a danger to their livers with long-term or frequent use. Baby drugs are so safe that most paediatricians will happily administer them to their own children very freely.

Having said that, it is vital to follow dosage guidelines on the packets because giving your baby an extra dose by mistake is dangerous. If this ever happens, perhaps if both you and your partner give your child medicine without consulting each other, then call NHS direct – 0845 4647, www.nhsdirect.nhs.uk. They will ask questions about your baby's weight and how much medicine he has had, then calculate the toxicity levels for his size and whether or not he is in danger.

The only potential problem with being too liberal in giving your baby painkillers is that it can mask more serious problems. So if your baby needs medicine for more than three days, see your doctor to eliminate any serious problems. Infant paracetamol is generally recommended for babies from two months, around the time of their first immunisations, and infant ibuprofen from three months. The infant forms of these two drugs are liquid, sweet-tasting and specially dilute for babies. It's certainly an advantage having these two baby painkillers to hand because you can actually use them both together. They work in different ways, and combined will work in synergy to give a super-powerful but safe painkilling effect which is useful for those occasions when your child is teething, or has some other very painful condition such as earache or tonsillitis. So it's okay to give the recommended dose of each painkiller at the same time when your baby needs a particularly strong painkilling effect. You can also alternate the two painkillers to avoid exceeding the dosage allowed in 24 hours for each drug.

Most babies will hate medicine until they are about 10 months, when they will start to gulp down the sweet, child-friendly flavours with gusto. But in the meantime it's best to forget about trying to use medicine spoons and buy a syringe from your pharmacy. Infant Neurofen comes with its own syringe, which is ideal. Use the syringe to squirt medicine to the back of your baby's throat, aiming for one side to avoid any gagging. Either swaddle your baby's arms or get your partner to hold them and be firm, decisive and quick. There isn't a nice way to give a reluctant baby medicine, but he certainly won't appreciate you being slow and dragging out the torment.

SLEEP

Total sleep required: 14–16 hours a day
Pattern: aim for your baby to have eight hours of uninterrupted sleep at night, for him to go to bed early, and to have two to three daytime naps

Dropping a nap

Your baby is likely to drop his late afternoon nap around now, having just two sleeps during the day – one in the morning and another at lunchtime. You'll notice that on some days he needs his final nap, and on others he doesn't fall asleep. Follow your baby's pattern because it will take him a couple of weeks to adjust to his new napping schedule. Ensure that there is a gap of at least three hours between your baby waking from his final nap and going to bed.

Foods to help your baby sleep better at night

At around the same time, your baby is likely to drop a milk feed, particularly if he is having two solid meals a day. Hopefully he'll be less hungry at night and drop a night feed. The jury is out over whether giving your baby solids helps get him through the night – plenty of mums say that it definitely makes a difference and that their baby dropped a night feed, but many experts say that milk alone is enough to get your baby through the night because weight for weight it contains more calories.

What you can be sure about is that some foods will be more conducive to sleep than others. Obviously if a certain food gives your baby indigestion it will keep him awake at night because wind or tummy ache will cause him to wake fully during his light sleep phase. So avoid giving him foods in the evening that seem to upset him, and over the coming weeks don't give him beans, lentils, onions or cabbage before bedtime as these all cause wind.

It's also important to give your baby foods that release energy slowly as these will keep his blood sugar stable and help him to feel full for longer. Such foods include sweet potato, pears, apples, peaches and carrots, which all have a low glycaemic index, meaning that they release sugar slowly. Whereas potatoes, pumpkin, parsnips, rice and papaya all have a high glycaemic index as they release sugar quickly, leaving your baby with an energy dip after a few hours. Interestingly, milk has a very low glycaemic index, suggesting that it does indeed sustain your baby for hours.

FEEDING

Total milk required: 600–1200 ml/20–40 oz a day (up to 240 ml/8 oz per feed)
Pattern: 4–6 feeds, plus solids – two cubes of purée twice a day
Weaning: continue with easy-to-digest fruit and vegetable purées: puréed courgette, potato and sweet potato. You can also try banana, papaya and avocado, which don't need to be cooked, just mashed
Weaning list so far: baby rice, carrot, pear, squash, pumpkin, apple and parsnip

This week we've expanded our list of purées, so continue to select different foods every few days as you encourage your baby to try lots of flavours. Because potato, sweet potato and banana are stodgier than the other foods listed, you may have to add extra breast milk or formula. We'll repeat the same list next week, so there's no need to rush your baby through the different tastes – take your time over the next few weeks and months.

You'll probably notice that your baby likes some foods more than others. It's fine to give him his favourites more often, but don't give up on the other foods – sometimes you have to offer a baby or toddler the same food 20 times before he will suddenly decide to eat it. And your main aim at the moment is to expose your baby to lots of different tastes rather than 'feeding him up' as he will still be getting nearly all of his nourishment from milk. Give your baby additional tastes, by mixing a couple of different fruits or vegetables together. You could also try adding soft herbs such as basil or coriander – cook and grind these in with your vegetable purées.

DEVELOPMENT AND PLAYING

Your baby will start to suck his feet when you change him, now that he is able to hold objects in two hands.

From this week onwards, your baby may roll from his back to his front. He's more likely to do this if he's good at rocking from side to side while on his back and if he can already roll from his front to his back. But don't be disappointed if your baby doesn't roll for another couple of months as it requires a lot of skill. He'll need both strength and coordination to swing his hips to one side while arching backwards as he tries to keep one arm out of the way and uses the other arm to add to the momentum of the roll.

Once your baby is able to roll on to his tummy you should still put him to sleep on his back to reduce his risk of cot death, and turn him back over should you notice that he wriggles on to his front in his sleep. Don't get too paranoid about him rolling on to his front though, as his risk of cot death is tiny now that he is five months old. Once he reaches eight months his risk is so minimal that you no longer need to worry about rolling him back.

WHEN TO SEE A DOCTOR

Head injury

Accidentally dropping your baby or letting him roll off a bed or changing table is extremely common, particularly around now when your baby is becoming mobile. If your baby falls he will probably hit his head and this can be very distressing, although hopefully not serious.

You don't need to take him to the doctor if his fall is less than two feet, the surface on which he fell is carpet or something soft, he cries straight away but then recovers within about 10 minutes, and your instinct says that he seems perfectly fine.

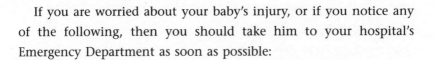

If you are worried about your baby's injury, or if you notice any of the following, then you should take him to your hospital's Emergency Department as soon as possible:

- **If he doesn't cry immediately, as this suggests that he was knocked out.**
- **If he vomits, as this indicates brain damage, although many babies will vomit once or twice after a minor injury too.**
- **If he's still miserable or irritable two hours later.**
- **If you can feel a swelling and are concerned.**
- **Definitely take your baby in if he has a 'boggy swelling', which feels soft and wet. This indicates a fractured skull – a crack in the bone causes immediate inflammation and this should be treated in hospital as an emergency.**

WHAT'S HAPPENING TO MUM

Your period may return about now if you are breastfeeding, although some women don't start menstruating until later. After giving birth, menstruation is usually heavier but less painful.

Being a new mum can be very sociable, as you spend your days drinking coffee with other mums and chatting about your babies. But sometimes it can be quite lonely – not everyone gets themselves enmeshed in a cosy social group of mums; you might have moved recently, or perhaps you were working right up until you gave birth.

There are plenty of groups out there, however. Try local playgroups (many GP surgeries and health centres have these) – there's often an area for babies to play safely away from feuding toddlers. Or you could sign up for a mums and babies yoga or swimming class – ask at your local sports centre.

You only need to find yourself one group, then things will quickly snowball as everyone will know what else is going on in your area.

PLANNING AHEAD
Buy a recipe book

In another month your baby will be old enough to eat meat, fish, dairy products and wheat, as well as being able to cope with finger foods and 'lumps'. This will make his diet a lot more interesting so you could choose a baby recipe book to give you interesting meal ideas, plus it may give you more purée ideas.

week 21

As you continue to wean your baby, it's essential to remember that it's not a race. Just as you followed your baby's lead when he was newborn and first started drinking milk, it's important to follow his lead now. Let your baby tell you how quickly to progress with solid food. If he reacts to a particular food, for example he may have mild diarrhoea, stop giving it or any new foods for a few days. This will delay his weaning programme, but that's not important. Never force your baby to eat – if he's not hungry then back off even if you've spent time fiddling around with small cubes of purée only to have to throw them away.

The best way to encourage your baby to eat solids is for the family to eat together – sitting down with other people for a meal is the most natural way for a baby to learn. And try sharing food with him (as long as it's from the weaning lists), for example you could let him have a suck of a pear or banana. He'll be delighted to eat 'adult' food.

Don't get frustrated and anxious on the days when your baby seems inexplicably disinterested in food – just remember that the long-term goal is to teach your child to enjoy food. Being anxious will generally have adverse effects. Try to stay relaxed when you feed your baby.

SLEEP

Total sleep required: 14–16 hours a day
Pattern: aim for your baby to have eight hours of uninterrupted sleep at night, for him to go to bed early, and to have two to three daytime naps

Sleep deprivation will really be taking its toll by now if your baby isn't a good sleeper; five months of broken nights will have left you feeling edgy, irritable and probably quite depressed. But there's a chance that your behaviour is contributing to your baby's sleep problem and stopping him from sleeping well by himself.

If you feel very anxious it actually makes the problem worse because babies pick up on tension and this can make them restless. So it's essential that you are calm and confident that your baby will sleep well because this will be reflected in your body language.

Try to isolate when you are at your most stressed – this is quite likely to be at your baby's bedtime, then arrange for your partner or someone else to be around. Getting some help for just a few days could break your anxiety cycle – you'll learn to cope better at the trickier times during the day and as you relax, your baby will too.

And the best quick fix for stress is exercise. So load up that buggy with shopping, push it up some hills, and walk a bit faster – once your heart is pounding and you feel out of breath, your stress hormone levels will fall.

Your baby's sleeping regime may also be hindered if you are clinging on to his infant stage and don't want him to grow up too quickly. Most mums would be quick to deny this as nonsense, saying that they are desperate to get their baby sleeping through the night, but an honest reappraisal may reveal that there is some truth in this, particularly if you know that you won't be having any more babies. Ask yourself if you are treasuring those moments in the middle of the night when you cuddle up with your baby, and if you really need to respond instantly to his cries or if you could perhaps leave him for a few minutes to settle himself. Of course, if you are happy attending to your baby throughout the night and genuinely relish this stage, then there's nothing fundamentally wrong with this – your baby certainly won't lose out by having the extra attention.

FEEDING

Total milk required: 600–1200 ml/20–40 oz (up to 240 ml/8 oz per feed)
Pattern: 4–6 feeds, plus solids – two to three cubes of purée twice a day
Weaning: continuing with easy-to-digest fruit and vegetable purées mentioned in previous weeks (see pages 234 and 242)
Weaning list so far: baby rice, carrot, pear, squash, pumpkin, apple, parsnip, courgette, potato, sweet potato, banana, papaya and avocado

Continue to work your way through the above fruit and vegetable list that we introduced last week to teach your baby about new tastes. He will probably be more proficient and eating larger quantities by now, but don't be surprised if your baby suddenly refuses a meal. Babies stop eating for a number of reasons, and as long as he is drinking well and not weeing any less than usual, there is no need to worry. Continue to offer him food then clear it away if he's not interested.

Reasons your baby might not eat

The most likely reason is that he has a cold, which quite often begins with a sore throat. There may not be any obvious cold symptoms, such as a runny nose, to begin with which is why it's important to trust that your baby really doesn't want any solid food at the moment and not to pressurise him. You may see an increase in his appetite once the cold breaks out. Other illnesses could also stop your baby wanting to eat, so keep a close eye on him and check his temperature if you think he might be unwell.

Teething will also put your baby off food because pressure on his gums will cause pain. If you are sure this is the cause of his loss of appetite, you could give him infant paracetamol (Calpol) 20 minutes before his meal as this should make a dramatic difference to his feeding.

Not being hungry or feeling tired will also reduce your baby's appetite, so work out whether he's due for a sleep, slept badly the previous night, or has recently had a milk feed and so is feeling full.

He may be a night feeder and drink milk throughout the night for comfort, and then not be very interested in food during the day (see page 187). This generally happens to breastfed babies who are sharing their parents' bed. If you've tried to resolve this problem and not had any luck, then it's time to get tough. Don't feed your baby after 3am and then by 7am, four hours later, he'll be keen to have his breakfast. It may take a couple of days to establish his daytime appetite, and there will be some crying in the small hours of the morning, but this feeding pattern needs addressing particularly as your baby is approaching six months when he will begin to get more of his calories and nutrients from solids, and less from milk.

DEVELOPMENT AND PLAYING

Your baby can play in an indoor baby harness swing, or baby bouncer, from around now. These are like swings that hang from elastic and are suspended from a doorway – your baby is strapped into a harness which allows him to stand and jump. He'll soon learn to bounce, turn around and spin, and he'll enjoy his new mobility as he builds his leg muscles. Just let him bounce for five minutes at first, and gradually build up to 20 minutes if he's happy. And of course, if your baby starts grizzling then take him out immediately because he's probably tired.

So far, your baby has probably been flat on his back in a pram or buggy when you've taken him out. But he's now old enough and has enough strength and head control to start sitting up and enjoying his surroundings. Prop him up when he's awake, and tip him back when it's time to sleep.

By now, your baby will be able to sit up by himself for a few seconds and will enjoy playing this 'balancing' game. Surround him with cushions and help him to sit by himself until he topples over – he'll love it. Don't leave him unattended.

!SAFETY TIP OF THE WEEK!
Don't add cereal to your baby's bottle

Well-meaning older relatives may suggest that you add baby cereal to your baby's bottle to thicken up his milk and help him to sleep better at night. You shouldn't do this because it will fill him up quickly and he may not take in enough fluid, putting him at risk from dehydration.

WHEN TO SEE A DOCTOR

Urinary tract infection

Urinary tract infection in babies is serious and needs to be assessed urgently by a doctor. The most obvious symptoms are vomiting and a fever, and you may notice strong, fishy smelling urine. Your doctor should refer your baby to hospital to arrange tests to pick up any abnormalities that he may have been born with, and also to see if he has developed kidney scars. Damaged kidneys can cause high blood pressure and even kidney failure later in life, which is why urgent medical treatment is so important. Hospital tests will also check for underlying problems with your baby's renal tract. Doctors will check the size, shape and position of the kidneys, and also look for vesicoureteric reflux,

VUR, which is when urine flows in the wrong direction from the bladder to the kidneys. This is, however, extremely rare.

Baby boys who have a urinary tract infection will ring more alarm bells than baby girls because they are less prone to this condition and it is more likely to be a sign of kidney problems.

Baby girls, on the other hand, are more susceptible to urinary tract infections so it's important to wipe them from front to back when changing their nappies to prevent bacteria getting from the bowel to the bladder.

WHAT'S HAPPENING TO MUM

No more excuses when it comes to exercise, unfortunately. Unless you have a particular injury or reason to avoid exercise, you can't use giving birth as a reason to be careful any more. You are physically ready to get out there and start training, hard. Of course from a fitness point of view you may need to build up gradually because, like anyone else, you will injure yourself if you try to do too much too soon. But as far as pregnancy hormones and loose ligaments are concerned – you're back to normal.

PLANNING AHEAD
High chairs

Buy a high chair because it won't be long before your baby is strong enough to sit in one. Unlike cots and car seats, it's okay to buy a second-hand high chair, although new ones start at about £25. As well as the look of the high chair, also consider how easy it is to clean and whether you can fold it away. Also, can you remove the tray and adjust the height so that your baby will be able to join you at the table when he is older, and how secure are the straps to keep him in? Remember that older babies and toddlers may try to escape from their high chairs.

week 22

It's quite likely that your baby will get his first tooth around now, in which case you may be wondering how to clean his teeth. The easiest way is to wipe the teeth with a damp cloth or cotton bud – don't use toothpaste at this age because your baby is too young to spit it out.

As well as wiping your baby's teeth, you can also buy a small, soft infant toothbrush and gently brush his teeth each evening. This is more to teach him lifelong good dental habits than to scrub away at any plaque. Keep brushing time short so that your baby doesn't become distressed, and combine it with wiping his teeth. Once he has his molars, or back teeth, you can just brush and stop using the cloth.

You'll soon discover just how difficult it can be to clean your baby's teeth, which is why it's important to prevent decay in the first place. Here's how to protect your baby's teeth. Firstly, babies shouldn't have any added sugar in their diet – it not only causes tooth decay but also gives them a sweet tooth. Another big no-no is going to sleep with a bottle of milk or juice in his mouth – your baby will nod off with a pool of sugary liquid around his teeth, which can result in decay. Breast milk is also sweet so if your baby shares your bed, don't let him feed on and off all night once he has teeth. Bottles of milk can cause damage during the day if your baby comfort sips for hours on end – one useful rule is not to allow him a bottle or cup in his pushchair as he'll end up having a drink that lasts on and off for well over an hour.

Of course tap water is harmless to teeth and can be drunk any time, but juice is even worse than milk because it's acidic and more sugary – even pure fruit juice that is diluted is harmful. Don't give juice to your baby and he won't develop a taste for it.

Finally, unless your baby comfort sucks on bottles and baby cups beyond the age of 18 months, there is no need to visit a dentist until he is five. But take him to the dentist sooner than this if you see anything obviously wrong such as brown marks on the teeth which might be cavities.

SLEEP

Total sleep required: *14–16 hours a day*
Pattern: *aim for your baby to have 8–12 hours of uninterrupted sleep at night, for him to go to bed early, and to have two to three daytime naps*

Some babies will sleep, uninterrupted, for 12 hours at night by this age but don't worry if your baby isn't doing this yet. You're definitely in the majority, and if you keep working at your baby's sleep patterns you will get there eventually. Throughout the book we've said that there are no quick fixes for getting your baby to sleep, but there are one or two things you can try which might help your baby to feel a little more sleepy at night.

Firstly, ensure that your baby has enough physical and mental exercise during the day, otherwise he may feel restless at bedtime. Swimming is a great way to exercise babies at this age as they are too young to crawl. It's worth calling your local pool to check on suitable times as some pools turn the temperature up for parent and baby sessions. Alternatively you could enrol your child in a parent and baby swimming class, which has an element of structure although it's still based on having fun (see page 198).

Whichever you choose, he'll love splashing and kicking and will be noticeably tired afterwards. Swimming will also stimulate your baby mentally because of the excitement of being in such a new and invigorating environment.

You can also encourage your baby to move and kick more during the day by giving him lots of time on a play mat rather than keeping him in his buggy or car seat for too long. Spend time playing with him and showing him lots of brightly coloured toys and other interesting objects – simple activities such as kicking at or crumpling newspaper will give your baby great pleasure.

Spending time with other people will also stimulate your baby – grandparents will have songs to sing him and he'll enjoy different voices and faces. Even taking him out on a train, bus or car will excite your baby if it's not something you do routinely.

Another activity you can try is massaging your baby as part of his bedtime routine – research at Miami University found that massaged babies wake less frequently during the night and cry less. The study found that stroking didn't have any of these benefits, but massaging with just enough pressure to indent the skin was effective. Use olive oil and make sure your baby is warm enough by bundling him up in towels, then gently massage his arms, legs and tummy. Then turn him over and massage his back and shoulders. Five minutes is long enough for your baby's first massage and just massaging his legs will probably be fine the first time. It'll take a few sessions to build up to a full body massage as your baby will have to get used to the new sensations. As always, respond to what your baby is 'telling' you – he will have preferences, so for example he might not want his tummy to be massaged. And be aware that some babies don't like being massaged at all, in which case don't do it.

FEEDING

Total milk required: *600–1200 ml/20–40 oz a day (up to 240 ml/8 oz per feed)*
Pattern: *4–6 feeds, plus solids – two to three cubes of purée three times a day*
Weaning: *difficult-to-digest fruit and vegetables: puréed broccoli, cauliflower, cabbage, leeks, green beans and peas, mashed raspberries, plus peeled and mashed peaches and nectarines, citrus fruit including oranges, plus lemon and lime juice which can be added to other fruit purées*
Weaning list so far: *baby rice, carrot, pear, squash, pumpkin, apple, parsnip, courgette, potato, sweet potato, banana, papaya and avocado*

Your baby is probably ready for three meals a day by now but, as always, follow his lead. You may notice that he wants less milk than he used to and he may drop another feed – again follow his lead although don't cut milk feeds to fewer than four over 24 hours because milk is still your baby's main source of nutrients and calories.

To keep your baby's diet varied you can now introduce almost any fruit or vegetable as long as it's puréed or mashed and easy to swallow.

The fruit and vegetables listed above are a little more difficult to digest than those previously listed – the vegetables are more likely to cause wind, and the fruit is more acidic, which can upset a baby's digestive systems. When introducing all new foods, watch your baby's reaction closely for a few days.

Give your baby oranges as juice rather than as a purée, but feed him this on a spoon rather than in a cup or a bottle to avoid establishing a sweet drink habit. Try adding squeezed juice to purées or fruit mashes, for example mix a little lime, lemon or orange juice with some mashed banana.

DEVELOPMENT AND PLAYING

Lots of babies are able to roll competently enough to be able to move across a room. So clear some space as your baby begins to get on the move.

Changing your baby's nappy will be difficult from now onwards as he becomes increasingly wriggly, kicking his legs and grabbing the nappy bag and cream. To distract him, try putting an unbreakable mirror next to his changing table – he'll be fascinated by the 'other baby' and this will make changing his nappy easier.

Your baby's short-term memory is only a few seconds long at the moment, which means that he soon forgets and cheers up if you take away a toy or leave the room. His long-term memory is more developed and he can now remember a toy that he saw two days ago – some experts think that babies of this age have memories that last 10 days. A more developed long-term memory enables your baby to feel comforted by the familiarity of his world – seeing the same people and surroundings from day to day.

Your baby continues to be fascinated by your face and will now start to touch it – putting his fingers in your mouth and nose, pulling your hair and trying to poke your eyes. This is a great game for your baby and he isn't trying to annoy or hurt you, even if he is quite rough sometimes. There's no point in trying to tell him not to be rough because babies don't understand the word 'no' before they're 10 months old.

WHEN TO SEE A DOCTOR

Glue ear

Although glue ear generally affects toddlers, it can also affect babies. It's important that it's picked up quickly because if hearing is impaired your baby's language development will be delayed. Your baby is more likely to suffer if he has a cleft palate, or if you or your partner are smokers. But glue ear can affect any baby and occurs when the Eustachian tube, which connects the middle ear to the back of the throat, becomes blocked. This results in sticky fluid blocking the middle ear, which makes hearing difficult. It can also cause pain.

If your baby seems in pain and rubs his ears, or if he doesn't seem to hear you as well as previously, you should get him checked by a doctor. Other clues include if he doesn't wake up so easily if you make a noise, if he doesn't turn round to hear who has entered a room, or if he doesn't babble in response to you talking to him. Your doctor will examine your baby's ear and will arrange to have his hearing checked, then if your baby isn't in pain, it will be a waiting game to see if the glue ear clears up by itself – this happens in nearly all cases but can take months.

If there isn't an improvement within three months, your doctor may refer your baby to an ear, nose and throat specialist, who might put him on a course of steroid nasal drops. Should there still be a problem when your child is between the age of one and two, he may have minor surgery to insert grommets – tiny plastic tubes that pierce the ear drum and release pressure, thus improving hearing. Grommets usually drop out within 6–18 months, after which your baby's glue ear will hopefully be cured. The operation is done under general anaesthetic as a day case.

WHAT'S HAPPENING TO MUM

You've no doubt been longing for an unbroken night's sleep, but when your baby finally sleeps through, you may be surprised to find that you don't sleep very well. This is quite common among mothers and happens because your body clock has been re-set to sleep in short bursts, so it will take a bit of time to adjust. But as your baby becomes better at sleeping through the night, you'll soon learn to sleep soundly again too. Before you know it, those endless sleepless nights will be a distant memory.

PLANNING AHEAD
Trial run of childcare

A lot of women go back to work after six months, and if this is what you intend then arrange for a trial run of your proposed childcare over the next couple of weeks. Even a couple of mornings a week at the new nursery or with the childminder will help your baby get used to the different arrangement, as well as give you confidence that things are going to work out.

week 23

One of the most controversial issues in baby care is controlled crying – leaving your baby to cry as you attempt to train him to sleep through the night. Some experts say that this is cruel and makes your baby stop trusting you, while others claim it is a tried and tested method of sleep training that is quick and effective. Both schools of thought are right up to a point. Deliberately leaving a very young baby to cry for long periods can be potentially dangerous because not feeding a baby who is younger than five months can lead to dehydration, particularly if your baby is small for his age. Also you won't be as practised at understanding your baby's cries while he is still very young so you are less likely to recognise genuine distress or pain.

But controlled crying can be an option once your baby is between five months and a year (when babies reach one they become a lot more stubborn and will cry for longer.) We want to emphasise that while this is a quick and effective sleep training method, it is also a last resort and we hope that most people reading this book won't have to endure this harrowing process.

Of course we would recommend starting with the more gentle approach of sleep training explained in this book – gradually giving your baby less and less 'help' getting to sleep. For many parents and babies this will work extremely well, although it can take several months to get your baby sleeping through the night.

But for some parents, there may come a moment when you simply can't stand broken nights any more. If this sounds like you then controlled crying, which takes about three nights, may be the answer. Once you are confident that your baby no longer 'needs' milk in the night, even though he may want it, there's nothing unkind about controlled crying. In fact, your baby's total crying time with this short, sharp method will be less than if you implement a gentler approach involving small bouts of crying over several months.

SLEEP

Total sleep required: *14–16 hours a day*
Pattern: *aim for your baby to have 8–12 hours of uninterrupted sleep at night, for him to go to bed early, and to have two to three daytime naps*

Should you decide to try controlled crying then it will take three nights, four at the most, to get a result. Your baby will probably cry for at least an hour. And he may cry for even longer on the second night than the first, but you should see an improvement on night three.

If your baby is used to feeding throughout the night, then you could use controlled crying for just one of his wake-up sessions at a time. You could start with bedtime, leaving him to cry himself to sleep. Then once your baby is able to settle himself at bedtime you could start to cut out his feeds one at a time by, again, using the controlled crying method. This drags the process out but may be easier for you and your baby to cope with – also you'll find that your baby will learn more quickly as you progress, and so cry for less time.

Why do it

Months of sleep deprivation have left you fearing for your relation-ship, your sense of humour and your sanity – it's been shown that mothers who aren't sleeping at night are more prone to post-natal depression (see page 93). Your health may also have been affected, and you'll be so exhausted that you're always snapping at people, particularly your partner. You feel too tired to be a good parent during the day because you don't have the energy to giggle and have fun with your baby, let alone take him out. You've tried the gentle method of sleep training but it doesn't seem to be working for your baby. You probably feel desperate.

Choose a good time

You'll need three or four nights when both you and your partner are prepared to be up in the night and tired the next day. Pick a time when you haven't got other worries and make sure that you and your partner agree on the plan – you'll both feel very stressed as your baby howls the night away and are likely to argue if one of you decides not to proceed.

Warn the neighbours

If neighbours know that this crying will only be for a few nights they will be tolerant and you won't be worrying about disturbing them during the night.

Check your baby is well

Ensure that your baby isn't ill. If your baby is coming down with a cold or has teething pain, then leaving him to cry by himself would be unkind – babies, just like adults, need extra fuss and love when they are unwell. So watch your baby closely during the day and make sure that he is his usual self. You could also take his temperature at bedtime just to be on the safe side – it should be under 38°C/100.4°F.

Fill his tummy

Make sure that his last feed is a big one and that, if you are breast-feeding, you're not short of milk. You'll know by now when your baby has had plenty of milk and is satisfied because he'll probably seem quite dopey.

Change his nappy

Don't wake your baby to change him, but ensure that his nappy is clean when you put him to bed and that you put on plenty of nappy cream to protect his skin in case he does a poo while he's crying.

Make his cot safe

Remove toys, blankets, mobiles and cot bumpers so that there is nothing he can get himself caught in. A baby sleeping bag is the best bedding option because it will stay on when he wriggles.

Once you've made your decision, there's no going back

The worst thing you can do if you go down the controlled crying route is to let your baby cry for 25 minutes then decide that you can't stand another minute, and that you have to put an end to this cruel nonsense and go and comfort him. This will give your baby a clear message that crying for 25 minutes makes mum appear and give him milk. If you do give in, you certainly won't be the first parent to have done so and if you still want to continue the controlled crying method then of course you can. However, it may take even more resolve next time as your baby will now be that little bit more determined, knowing that crying gets him rescued.

Going into his room while he is crying

Some experts suggest going in to your baby every five minutes because he'll feel comforted when he sees you. Plenty of parents have found this to be an effective, but less harsh, way of sleep training. In our experience, if you've reached the point where you feel you need to do controlled crying, your baby will probably be very used to getting a lot of attention throughout the night. So we think you'll probably need a more drastic version of controlled crying to break the pattern. We've found that going in every five minutes can seem like teasing to some babies who will be frantic to be lifted out of the cot, and will then become more upset than ever when they realise this isn't going to happen as they watch you leave the room. So staying out of the room actually works better for some babies and is the method often advised at sleep clinics, where they see the most desperate cases of baby-sleep problems. Our advice is to check on your baby without him seeing you – perhaps through a crack in the door.

While he is crying

Your baby will by turns scream in rage or whimper pitifully, making you feel like a heartless parent with no nurturing instincts. Remind yourself that he isn't hungry, that he has a clean nappy and he isn't ill or in pain. Keep an eye on the clock so that when an hour has passed you'll know that the end is near – also it will help you know what to expect over the next couple of nights. To help distract yourself from the crying you can try watching a DVD; this may help stop you from going in to your baby.

WHAT HIS CRIES SAY

Listen carefully to your baby's crying and ask yourself what he'd be saying if you could understand him. It would probably be something like, 'I'm furious. I want to get out of my cot, I want a drink of milk because that's what I'm used to, where are you – you're usually here by now? Can't you hear me? I'm going to cry even louder to make you come and get me.'

What he's probably not saying is, 'I'm terrified, I feel unloved and insecure, I'm feeling ill and in pain, I'm desperately hungry because I've gone much too long without milk, I'm all alone in the world, this is doing irreparable damage to me mentally, and I'm never going to forgive you.' Remind yourself that he's still a baby with very simple needs and he's not yet a complex teenager.

Be ready to change the bed

Very occasionally, babies cry so hard that they make themselves sick. Although this sounds absolutely terrible just remember that, unlike older children, babies don't feel upset if they are sick. To them it's just like weeing or pooing. It's also worth remembering that babies vomit very easily and if they bring up their milk through crying it doesn't mean they are in pain or ill. If your baby is sick, then this is about as tough as controlled crying gets and you will have to be strong minded not to scoop him into your arms to comfort him. But do try to resist as you'll only prolong the process and his misery. If you comfort him and decide to abandon controlled crying for the night but then decide to proceed a few days later your baby will feel utterly bewildered, and probably cry for longer than ever. It's actually kinder to have a spare sheet and baby wipes to hand, then clean your baby up as efficiently as you can without chatting to him. Just say, shhh go to sleep. As you change the sheet you can do half the cot at a time to avoid having to lift him out. Try to avoid giving your baby the message that he's going to be lifted out of his cot and fed.

The next day

Your baby will wake up refreshed, be as cuddly and loving as ever and behave as though nothing happened. You're bound to be feeling guilty, but see the programme through because you've made a decision to try controlled crying and it really won't do your baby any harm.

FEEDING

Total milk required: 600–1200 ml/20–40 oz a day
(up to 240 ml/8 oz per feed)
Pattern: 4–5 milk feeds, plus solids – three to four cubes of purée three times a day
Weaning: chicken, turkey, beef, pork and lamb
Weaning list so far: baby rice, carrot, pear, squash, pumpkin, apple, parsnip, courgette, potato, sweet potato, banana, papaya, avocado, broccoli, cauliflower, cabbage, leeks, green beans, peas, raspberries, peaches, nectarines, oranges, lemon juice and lime juice

Now that your baby is almost six months old, you can introduce him to meat. Begin with chicken, which is a little easier to digest than red meat, and make sure that it is ground up and puréed well. You might want to add water or formula milk to make it easier for your baby to swallow. Serve the chicken with vegetables and potato or sweet potato to make a balanced meal. If chicken proves a success, then try your baby on red meat, perhaps beginning with beef.

Meat is an excellent source of iron for babies and it's important that your baby gets this nutrient from now onwards. This is because babies are born with a store of iron, but this is depleted at around six months, which is why you should try to wean your baby on to meat quite quickly.

VEGETARIAN BABY

If you're giving your baby a vegetarian diet, then he can get his iron from pulses and green vegetables, as well as eggs. But iron isn't absorbed as easily from these sources as it is from meat, so do talk to your health visitor about your baby's diet. Vitamin C is particularly important for vegetarian babies as it helps the absorption of iron. Good sources include blueberries, kiwis, raspberries and citrus fruit.

Once your baby is six months, you will need to ensure that two of his meals a day include eggs or dairy products such as cheese or yoghurt so that he gets enough high-quality protein. Animal protein is the highest quality, followed by soya, which is the only plant protein to contain all the amino acids: feed tofu to your baby as it's bland and also has a very soft texture. Beans and lentils are also good plant sources of protein.

Instant baby food that doesn't come from a jar

If you find making purées too fiddly and time-consuming and have resorted to using jars of baby food, there are still plenty of meals that you can prepare yourself which take little effort.

- **Try finely mashed avocado, papaya, banana or peach – you can add a little baby milk and baby rice to these.**
- **A sweet potato can be microwaved for 10 minutes then the flesh mashed with a little olive oil.**
- **You can buy cubes of frozen chopped spinach which can be microwaved and mashed.**
- **Mashed tofu also works well, and so do mashed, tinned beans such as butter beans and chick peas – these are instant sources of protein that don't need cooking.**

As always, remember that if you are introducing your baby to a new food, wait a few days to ensure he isn't allergic to it.

DEVELOPMENT AND PLAYING

Your baby will be able to sit up by himself for about 10 seconds although he will probably be quite wobbly as his head is still big for his body, causing him to topple over. Make sure he's sitting on something soft, such as carpet, and that there's nothing hard that he may fall against. Over the next few weeks your baby will develop enough strength in his hips and spine to be able to sit for longer, enabling him to see easily around the room and play with toys.

Your baby is now able to grab moving objects and can work out how quickly and in what direction an object is moving so that he can swipe at it with his arm. Instead of moving with jerky movements, your baby moves his arms smoothly as he reaches for a toy. And he now has the dexterity to pass small objects from one hand to the other.

Your baby can now anticipate nice things that happen during his day such as bathtime. So he may kick his legs, shake his head and squeal when you carry him wrapped in a towel into the bathroom.

Although your baby can't talk, he's now very good at communicating. For example, he will hold out his arms to be picked up, cuddle you when he wants to stay with you, then arch his back when he wants to be put down.

For the last few weeks, your baby has been playing with his feet and is now starting to use them, along with his hands, to hold and explore toys – this is a short phase which he will outgrow within a month.

!SAFETY TIP OF THE WEEK!
Smoke alarms

You should already have fitted smoke alarms in your home to minimise the risk of being injured from a house fire, but if you haven't then it's vital you do so now. Babies are particularly vulnerable because they are immobile so can't escape from either smoke inhalation or from a fire.

It is advisable to install an alarm on each floor, with one in the hallway and one on each landing – making sure there's one outside your (and your baby's) bedroom. Your house or flat may benefit from other smoke alarms depending on its layout.

Smoke alarms come in two different types – ionisation and optical. Ionisation is the cheapest type (under £5) and is very sensitive to flaming fires (like a chip pan fire) while the optical version is more expensive but is good at detecting slow-burning fires, such as smouldering furniture. You can also buy combined versions for about £15, which offer the best of both worlds.

Whatever alarm you choose, or even if your home already has alarms, make sure a working battery is fitted and try to test the alarm every week. Every year people die from smoke inhalation in house fires after removing the smoke alarm battery to use in something else and then forgetting to replace it.

It's also a good idea to have a fire escape plan worked out so that you and your partner know exactly what to do if the worst happens – you need to be able to exit your home with your baby as quickly and safely as possible. For more information on smoke alarms, as well as lots of great advice on fire prevention, log on to www.firekills.co.uk.

WHEN TO SEE A DOCTOR

Flattened head syndrome

This condition occurs when your baby's soft skull becomes flattened from hours of lying on his back and it is becoming increasingly common now that parents put their babies to sleep on their backs to avoid cot death (see page 28). You may notice that your baby also gets a bald patch on the back of his head from so much time spent lying on his back. The side of your baby's skull can also become misshapen if he likes to lie with his head to one side, resulting in a wonky shaped head known as plagiocephaly (see opposite).

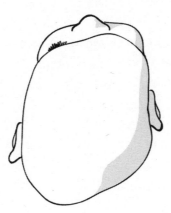

Your baby's soft skull can become wonky from hours of lying with his head to one side – a condition known as plagiocephaly.

You can tilt his head gently to the other side to correct this, although he will probably shuffle back into his favourite sleeping position again. You can also reverse his position on his changing mat so that he looks at you on the opposite side – this will help to reduce any flattening of the side of his head. Spending plenty of time on his front when he is awake will also help to minimise any further misshaping of your baby's head.

In minor cases of flattened head syndrome and plagiocephaly, the problem will right itself once your baby starts sitting up and spends less time on his back. Some babies, however, will grow up with a slightly misshapen skull but this is nothing to worry about because the only problem is cosmetic and once your baby's hair grows, it will be barely noticeable. If you are concerned, then see your doctor for reassurance.

WHAT'S HAPPENING TO MUM

For the first year of your baby's life you are entitled to free dental treatment, so book yourself an appointment if you haven't seen your dentist recently. There's a reasonable chance that you will need treatment for a number of reasons. Firstly, your dentist would have done the minimum amount of treatment while you were pregnant and you may not have had x-rays, which means that you could well have a few undiscovered cavities that need filling. And as a new mum you will have been struggling to get dressed in the morning let alone managing to floss and carefully brush your teeth twice a day. You may well have indulged in lots of sugary foods and drinks while pregnant. Finally, if you are breastfeeding, then you shouldn't use fluoride mouthwash so you won't have as much protection against decay.

PLANNING AHEAD
Buy child-proof safety devices

From around now you will have to think about making your home safe. As well as taking common-sense measures such as moving easy-to-grab heavy ornaments, you'll need to buy stair gates, drawer locks and plastic covers for plug sockets. You may also need a fire guard, door stops to prevent doors being slammed, and corner covers for sharp furniture. You can buy child safety equipment from baby shops and also from DIY stores, but allow time for shopping around as it takes a while to find everything that you need.

week 24

Congratulations! Your baby will be six months old at the end of this week, and he now eats solid food, can nearly sit up, is thinking about crawling and doesn't always resort to howling when he wants to communicate.

Your baby's growth and development over the last six months has been phenomenal, but this is only the beginning. By the end of his first year your baby will be crawling, clapping, waving, sitting in a high chair and sharing family meals. He might even be starting to walk, or perhaps he'll say a word or two.

You can expect your child to continue to baffle and confuse you for many years and there will always be days when it all seems too much. But you're not alone, as you'll discover when you talk to other parents. Don't forget that your health visitor and GP will always be on hand to help and advise, or to refer you to a range of experts including behavioural psychologists, sleep specialists, dietitians, speech therapists and physiotherapists.

If you're ever seriously worried about your child, don't hesitate to see your doctor for an emergency appointment – or even go to your hospital's Emergency Department. It takes doctors and nurses moments to make an assessment and they'd rather put your mind at rest than let a potentially seriously ill child miss out on medical care.

For parents, the first six months of your baby's life are exhilarating and exhausting in equal amounts, and it's no small achievement to have reached this huge milestone. From now on in, it does get easier in many ways – your child becomes more independent, less needy and more giving, although you'll still be the centre of his world for many, many years to come. The thrill of seeing him develop his own personality and character is one of the immeasurable joys of parenthood. So enjoy your baby to the full and relish wholeheartedly the opportunity and good fortune of being able to share his daily journey of wide-eyed exploration, as he grows into the confident, happy and capable child you have helped him become.

SLEEP

Total sleep required: *14–16 hours a day*
Pattern: *aim for your baby to have 8–12 hours of uninterrupted sleep at night, for him to go to bed early, and to have two to three daytime naps*

Throughout this book we've talked about how to get your baby to sleep well at night, but even if you've got an easy baby it's unlikely that he has a textbook sleeping pattern. Something as simple as getting a cold or a tooth coming through will guarantee a broken night. Disturbed sleep is an unavoidable part of being a parent and something that previous generations have struggled with just as much as today's mums and dads.

Next time you struggle out of bed to soothe your crying baby, console yourself with the fact that you are almost certainly doing better than our predecessors who, it turns out, resorted to using drugs and alcohol to soothe their children! In the 18th century mothers thought nothing of giving gin to a restless baby and would make it up into a sweet punch drink. Upper-class babies would have their dummies dipped in brandy. By the 19th century, solutions of opium were freely given to babies so that parents could get some sleep.

During the Industrial Revolution an 18-hour working day was the norm, so an opium mixture called 'Mother's helper' or 'Infant's quietness' would seem like a godsend to exhausted parents. And gripe water worked until the beginning of the last century because it contained alcohol – today's version does little to calm an upset baby.

You might think that drugging your baby to sleep is extreme, but plenty of parents today buy baby medicines containing antihistamine, which has a sedating effect. These are available over the counter and licensed for babies from three months old, but we don't recommend them as sleep aids because they won't treat the underlying problem.

A shocking number of parents find it amusing to give their child alcohol, and hope that it will calm them and aid sleep. But this is extremely dangerous because alcohol has a potent effect on a baby's blood sugar levels making him severely hypoglycaemic and putting him at risk of going into a coma and even dying. So don't ever be tempted to give your baby even a small amount of alcohol from your finger.

There aren't any shortcuts to teaching your child to sleep through the night. It's a slog and if you're not making progress and find that nothing you do seems to work, then you could talk to your GP or health visitor about getting a referral to an NHS sleep clinic. You'll get lots of support, plus guidance on how to teach your baby to become a good sleeper for life.

FEEDING

Total milk required: 600–1200 ml/20–40 oz a day
(up to 240 ml/8 oz per feed)
Pattern: 4–5 feeds, plus solids – around four to five cubes of purée three times a day
Weaning: wheat, fish, eggs and dairy products to be introduced over the next few weeks
Weaning list so far: baby rice, carrot, pear, squash, pumpkin, apple, parsnip, courgette, potato, sweet potato, banana,

*papaya, avocado, broccoli, cauliflower, cabbage, leeks, green
beans, peas, raspberries, peaches, nectarines, oranges, lemon
juice, lime juice, chicken, turkey, beef, pork and lamb*

This is the final week of our weaning programme, although the
weaning process continues well into your baby's first year. But for
now, we get your baby started on wheat and make suggestions for
the next few weeks, by which time he'll be eating a huge variety of
foods. This week, give your baby a baby cereal containing wheat that
is easy to swallow, or you could try mashed up Weetabix and formula
milk. Allow seven days to ensure that your baby shows no adverse
reaction to wheat before progressing with other foods.

Then move on to dairy products – you could start using a little
cows' milk in your cooking, or adding a cheese sauce or some plain
yoghurt to your baby's vegetables. Again, wait a week to ensure that
your baby is able to tolerate dairy products.

When you give your baby fish, choose a soft white fish to begin
with and remove all the bones – don't give your baby smoked fish
as it is too salty.

And, finally, you can give your baby eggs – begin with the yolk as
this is less likely to cause an allergic reaction than the egg white.
Always make sure that the egg yolk is hard-boiled to reduce the risk
of food poisoning.

A six-month-old baby's introduction to solids

If you waited until your baby is six months old to introduce solids,
there is no need to follow this weaning programme. In fact you'll
have to get your baby on to a variety of foods such as meat, wheat,
dairy and eggs as quickly as possible to ensure he has plenty of nutrients now that he's a bigger baby.

By all means use our programme as a general guide to get you
going. The baby rice is a great way to begin and this is the one part
of our programme we urge you not to rush (see page 219) because
your baby will need time to get used to having new textures in his

mouth and learning to swallow solid food. But once he progresses to puréed fruit and vegetables, you can speed up the weaning programme by offering him as many varieties as possible, ensuring that he gets meat within the first month because iron stores become depleted at around six months (see page 267).

Once you have worked through the weaning programme and your baby is happy eating meat, dairy products, wheat, fish and eggs, you can continue to introduce him to more unusual fruit and vegetables.

Foods unsuitable for a six-month-old

Although your baby can now eat a varied diet, there are still some foods he should avoid until he is older.

Lumpy foods

Avoid lumpy food until your baby is about seven months, after which you don't have to purée everything quite so finely. Then it will be okay for him to have small pieces of cooked vegetables in his purées, little bits of pasta, peas and so on. You can also start giving him finger foods at this age, such as pieces of cheese and toast to pick up and chew.

Pâté, unpasteurised soft cheese and shellfish

These can cause food poisoning so don't give them to your baby until he is at least one.

Honey

Wait until your baby is a year old because honey occasionally contains bacteria, which can cause infant botulism in the under-ones.

Salt

Don't add salt to your baby's food during his first year, then continue to keep him away from salt for as long as possible. Babies shouldn't get a taste for salt as this makes them more likely to get heart problems later in life. Also their kidneys are too immature to cope with

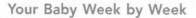

a high salt diet. Try to limit salty foods such as sausages and packet foods not aimed at babies.

Biscuits

Avoid sweet foods for as long as possible because added sugar will give your baby a sweet tooth.

Low-fat milk and cheese

Babies should eat full-fat products until they are at least two years old. They need the fat for brain development and it helps vitamin absorption.

Fibre

Babies shouldn't eat a high-fibre diet because the bulk fills them up and they eat less overall.

Nuts

Avoid giving your child whole nuts until he is five in case he chokes. Also see the allergy section opposite about giving your child peanut butter and ground nuts before then.

Whole grapes and cherries

Every year children choke to death on these fruits so cut them in half, or even quarters, and remove any stones until your child is five.

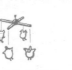

ALLERGIES

If there is a family history of food allergy, then take care when introducing cows' milk, wheat and eggs into your baby's diet as these are the foods most likely to cause allergies. Delaying the introduction of these foods until your baby is one is thought to reduce your baby's chance of developing an allergy. It's worth doing this if you have food allergies in your family.

If there is a family history of peanut allergy, hay fever, eczema or asthma then don't give your baby peanut butter or foods containing peanut oil until he is three. This will reduce his chance of developing such an allergy. But if there's no family history, your child can eat ground nuts from the age of six months.

Vitamin drops

If you are still breastfeeding, you could consider giving your baby vitamin drops to supplement his diet. This will ensure that he gets enough vitamin A and D, which some babies go short of. Babies who drink at least 600 ml/20 oz/a pint of formula milk a day don't need vitamin drops because formula milk is supplemented with vitamins. You will find infant vitamin drops at your pharmacist, and they are free until your child is five from your clinic if you are on income support.

279

DEVELOPMENT AND PLAYING

Babies start to crawl from between seven and ten months, and if your baby is going to be an early crawler then he will start to 'creep' around now. This is when he lies on his tummy and shunts himself along with his legs and arms. Encourage him by letting him shuffle on his tummy towards a toy.

If you play peekaboo with your baby he's now able to anticipate you saying 'boo' and will giggle as he waits. Previously he would have had no expectation because he hadn't developed 'object permanence' (see page 203). He thought that if he couldn't see someone or something it didn't exist. This new understanding means that he now looks for toys that he has dropped instead of assuming that they no longer exist.

Your baby can copy your facial expressions so have fun – try sticking your tongue out, blowing raspberries, and opening and closing your mouth like a fish.

As your baby's vision improves and he is able to see details, he will start to enjoy more complex toys, such as those with doors to open, buttons to press, handles to wind and dials to turn. You'll need to help him at first, and don't expect him to be able to concentrate for longer than a couple of minutes at this stage.

!SAFETY TIP OF THE WEEK!
Cover plug sockets

Your baby is becoming more mobile by the day so it's time to cover your plug sockets with plastic, childproof covers. You should also put a stair gate at the top of the stairs to stop him falling down – you don't need a guard at the bottom yet as he's still too young to crawl up by himself, although it won't be long.

WHEN TO SEE A DOCTOR

Chicken pox

Your baby will be protected against chicken pox until he is three months if you have had chicken pox yourself. This is due to the placental transfer of antibodies while you were pregnant and some of this protection will last until your baby is six months old. But from now onwards he will have no immunity to chicken pox and be vulnerable. The disease begins with a fever that is followed by a rash on the face and trunk that spreads to the arms and legs. The rash will blister within a few hours and be extremely itchy, but should calm down after four days.

You only need to see your doctor if you are unsure of the diagnosis, but, as always, go if you are worried about your baby. Your doctor will be able to do little apart from giving reassurance.

To help your baby, trim his nails to reduce the damage he does when he scratches, try to put him in scratch mittens, give him infant paracetamol or ibuprofen to bring his fever down and reduce discomfort, try a cool bath with bicarbonate of soda to relieve itching, and apply calamine lotion to the spots.

Although chicken pox is very unpleasant, your baby will only catch it once and you can feel glad that at least it's out of the way. Your baby won't be infectious five days after the first spots appeared, once the blisters have crusted over, and if he does pass it on, the other person won't develop chicken pox for at least 10 days.

WHAT'S HAPPENING TO MUM

Six months have passed since you gave birth and you'll have lost a lot of your baby weight and be looking more like a yummy mummy by the day! Although you're probably feeling back to your old self and have lots of energy, it can take a year before your body fully recovers from giving birth. In the meantime you may find that you are more susceptible to colds and other minor illnesses, particular if you start back at work – early nights and healthy living should definitely be on the agenda for the next six months to allow a full recovery.

Life will never be the same again now that you are a mum, but it's essential that you find time to enjoy yourself without your baby. Going out without him may feel strange but you'll quickly come to relish your free time. Don't feel in the slightest bit guilty because part of being a good mum is being happy and relaxed – so if you haven't found yourself a decent babysitter yet, start asking around.

PLANNING AHEAD
The future

Throughout this book, we've covered all sorts of practical suggestions in the Planning Ahead section to help you get organised with your new baby. From arranging child benefit to making sure you've got a good supply of teething gel, we've tried to ensure that you're always one step ahead of the game.

But as we leave you now with your six-month-old, it's almost impossible to plan so thoroughly for the future. Development, interests and physical needs will be completely different from child to child. You'll no doubt be inundated with well-intentioned advice over the coming months and years, but every baby – and every parenting experience – is unique. What works for other parents won't necessarily be best for you and your child – and it's this that makes having children such a challenge as well as a never-ending joy.

APPENDICES

weaning schedule
summary

The earliest that you can start your baby on solids is from the age of 17 weeks (four months), but many mums follow Department of Health and the World Health Organisation guidelines which recommend that mothers exclusively breastfeed for six months before introducing solids.

If you have left solids until your baby is six months old, you may want to progress more quickly through our weaning programme to ensure that he doesn't go short of important nutrients.

Don't rush the baby rice stage because your baby will need time to get used to having new textures in his mouth and learning to swallow solid food. Once he progresses to puréed fruit and vegetables, you can speed up the weaning programme by not offering your baby quite so many varieties before trying him on meat. Aim to give him meat a month after his first introduction to solid food – when he is seven months old. It is important to get his iron stores up, which, as mentioned last week, become depleted at around six months.

Once you have worked through the weaning programme and your baby is happy eating meat, dairy products, wheat, fish and eggs, you can continue to introduce him to more unusual fruit and vegetables so that he doesn't miss out.

Note: when we say 'milk' we are referring to breast milk or formula. We don't introduce cows' milk or other dairy products into our weaning schedule until the eighth week.

First week:
One teaspoon of baby rice mixed with milk once a day.

Your baby will probably spit most of this out because he's not used to solids and is happy to just feel the texture of food in his mouth.

Second week:
Two teaspoons of baby rice mixed with milk, plus a little puréed carrot or pear twice a day.

Your baby can experience new tastes this week. Once he is able to swallow a little rice, give him a few teaspoons of puréed carrot and if he shows no adverse reaction after three days, offer him pear. You can mix the purées with baby rice and milk to make it more familiar and also to bulk it out. You can continue to use baby rice throughout the weaning programme whenever you want to bulk a purée out.

Third week:
Two cubes of purée twice a day.

Try easy-to-digest fruit and vegetable purées: squash, pumpkin, apple and parsnip.

Weaning list so far – baby rice, carrot and pear.

You can start freezing vegetable and fruit purées in ice-cube trays, then give your baby two cubes at a time. Build up your baby's menu, introducing a new food every few days.

Fourth week:

Two cubes of purée twice a day.

And add puréed courgette, potato and sweet potato. You can also try banana, papaya and avocado, which don't need to be cooked, just mashed.

Weaning list so far – baby rice, carrot, pear, squash, pumpkin, apple and parsnip.

Fifth week:

Two to three cubes of purée twice a day.

Continue with easy-to-digest fruit and vegetable purées mentioned in previous weeks.

Weaning list so far – baby rice, carrot, pear, squash, pumpkin, apple, parsnip, courgette, potato, sweet potato, banana, papaya and avocado.

Sixth week:

Two to three cubes of purée three times a day.

Try giving your baby more difficult-to-digest fruit and vegetables including puréed broccoli, cauliflower, cabbage, leeks, green beans and peas. You can also try mashed raspberries, peeled and mashed peaches and nectarines, and citrus fruit including oranges, plus lemon and lime juice which can be added to other fruit purées.

Weaning list so far – baby rice, carrot, pear, squash, pumpkin, apple, parsnip, courgette, potato, sweet potato, banana, papaya and avocado.

Seventh week:
Three to four cubes of purée three times a day.

From this week you can start giving your baby chicken, turkey, beef, pork and lamb.

Once your baby is almost six months old, you can introduce him to meat. Begin with chicken, which is the easiest to digest, and make sure that it is ground up and puréed well. You can add water or formula milk to make it easier for your baby to swallow. You can serve meat with vegetables and potato or sweet potato for a balanced meal.

Weaning list so far – baby rice, carrot, pear, squash, pumpkin, apple, parsnip, courgette, potato, sweet potato, banana, papaya, avocado, broccoli, cauliflower, cabbage, leeks, green beans, peas, raspberries, peaches, nectarines, oranges, lemon juice and lime juice.

Eighth week:
Four to five cubes of purée three times a day.

Wheat, fish, eggs and dairy products can be introduced over the next few weeks.

You can give your baby a baby cereal containing wheat that is easy to swallow, or try mashed up Weetabix and formula milk. Allow seven days to ensure that your baby shows no adverse reaction to wheat, then move on to dairy products. You could start using a little cows' milk in your cooking, or adding cheese sauce or some plain yoghurt to your baby's vegetables. Again wait a week to ensure that your baby is able to tolerate dairy products.

When you give your baby fish, choose a soft white fish to begin with and remove all the bones – don't give your baby smoked fish as it is too salty.

And, finally, you can give your baby eggs – begin with the yolk as this is less likely to cause an allergic reaction than the egg white. Always make sure that the egg yolk is hard-boiled to reduce the risk of food poisoning.

Weaning list so far – baby rice, carrot, pear, squash, pumpkin, apple, parsnip, courgette, potato, sweet potato, banana, papaya, avocado, broccoli, cauliflower, cabbage, leeks, green beans, peas, raspberries, peaches, nectarines, oranges, lemon juice, lime juice, chicken, turkey, beef, pork and lamb.

useful addresses

NCT breastfeeding counsellors
Tel: 0300 330 0772
www.nct.org.uk

La Leche League
PO Box 29
West Bridgford
Nottingham
NG2 7NP
Tel: 0845 456 1855
www.laleche.org.uk

Medela
www.medela.com

Cry-sis
BM Cry-sis
London
WC1N 3XX
Tel: 08451 228 669
www.cry-sis.org.uk

Unicef
2 Kingfisher House
Woodbrook Crescent
Billericay
CM12 0EQ
Tel: 0844 801 2414
www.unicef.org.uk

Pregnancy and post-natal exercise:

www.postnatalexercise.co.uk

Child Benefit:

Inland Revenue
Tel: 0845 302 1444
www.hmrc.gov.uk/childbenefit

Child Tax Credit:

Inland Revenue
Tel: 0845 300 3900
www.hmrc.gov.uk/taxcredits

index

Baby Medical Conditions